Strokes

An Illustrated Guide to Brain Structure, Blood Supply, and Clinical Signs

James P. Bowman, PhD
Retired, The Chicago Medical School

Frank D. Giddings, MS, AMI
Retired, Director
Biomedical Communications
Colorado State University

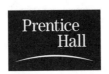

Prentice Hall

Upper Saddle River, New Jersey

Library of Congress Cataloging-in-Publication Data
Bowman, James P. (James Philip), (date)
    Strokes: an illustrated guide to brain structure,
blood supply, and clinical signs / James P. Bowman,
Frank D. Giddings.
        p.; cm.
    Includes bibliographical references and index.
    ISBN 0-13-048849-6
        1. Cerebrovascular disease. I. Title: Illustrated
guide to brain structure, blood supply, and clinical
signs. II. Giddings, Frank D., (date) III. Title.
        [DNLM: 1. Cerebrovascular Accident—diagnosis.
2. Cerebrovascular Accident—therapy. WL 355
B787s 2003]
    RC388.5.B66 2003
    616.8′1—dc21
                                            2002025796

Notice: The authors and the publisher of this volume have taken care that the information and technical recommendations contained herein are based on research and expert consultation, and are accurate and compatible with the standards generally accepted at the time of publication. Nevertheless, as new information becomes available, changes in clinical and technical practices become necessary. The reader is advised to carefully consult manufacturers' instructions and information material for all supplies and equipment before use, and to consult with a healthcare professional as necessary. This advice is especially important when using new supplies or equipment for clinical purposes. The authors and publisher disclaim all responsibility for any liability, loss, injury, or damage incurred as a consequence, directly or indirectly, of the use and application of any of the contents of this volume.

Publisher: Julie Levin Alexander
Executive Assistant: Regina Bruno
Acquisitions Editor: Mark Cohen
Assistant Editor: Melissa Kerian
Editorial Assistant: Mary Ellen Ruitenberg
Director of Manufacturing
  and Production: Bruce Johnson
Managing Editor: Patrick Walsh
Production Editor: Pat McCutcheon, WestWords, Inc.
Production Liaison: Cathy O'Connell
Manufacturing Buyer: Pat Brown
Design Director: Cheryl Asherman
Senior Design Coordinator: Maria Guglielmo
Composition: WestWords, Inc.
Printing and Binding: Phoenix Color/Book Tech Park

Pearson Education LTD.
Pearson Education Australia PTY, Limited
Pearson Education Singapore, Pte. Ltd
Pearson Education North Asia Ltd
Pearson Education Canada, Ltd.
Pearson Educación de Mexico, S.A. de C.V.
Pearson Education — Japan
Pearson Education Malaysia, Pte. Ltd

For Edie, Christy,
and stroke victims

CONTENTS

PREFACE

The impetus for this book arose after one of us (J.B.) suffered a stroke and, upon being discharged from the hospital, was given a thin binder containing material to "explain" what strokes were and how they might affect one's brain and behavior. The material was woefully inadequate. Because I am a professor of brain anatomy, my wife asked me, "Why don't you write one?" This book is the result. It represents the combined effort of a neuroanatomist and medical illustrator to present a visually compelling account of the blood supply of the brain, the brain areas affected by different types of strokes, and the resulting clinical signs observed in the patient.

It is difficult to imagine a structure that matches the human brain in complexity. However, this monograph is not a reference book and no effort has been made to introduce the basics of brain structure and function; nor is it intended to supplant longer, more comprehensive textbooks of neurology. The organizational plans assumed in textbooks on brain structure, function, or neurology are notably different from the plan we adopted. Nature dictates a major organizational theme: Namely, sets of brain structures are bound together by virtue of their being in the territory supplied by a given blood vessel. The number of such structures affected in a particular stroke in a given patent might vary depending upon the severity of the stroke and individual patient factors. But the potential array is stable except in massive and fatal strokes where the force of escaping blood dictates its own path of destruction. Given this fact of brain anatomy, it remains then to distinguish between the different types of cerebrovascular disease that can affect a given blood vessel and result in a stroke. Such disease processes are treated in Chapters 4 through 8 with Chapter 4 serving as the model for the remainder. The glossary was developed with an eye toward defining those terms physicians and other healthcare professionals might use in explaining patient status to patients or their families.

Two features contribute to this book's uniqueness. Many fine neurology texts contain more thorough descriptions of the brain pathophysiology, giving rise to the signs and symptoms associated with different types of strokes as well as treatment options. But as far as we are aware, none contain either the quality or density of illustrations presented in this book. The set of personal observations made by one of us as a consequence of having sustained a stroke is the second unique feature of this book. These insights are the subject of Chapter 2, and a number of the topics selected for coverage in Chapter 1 were chosen because of this experience. Many excellent autobiographical accounts, written by persons in the medical profession as well as laymen, describe the varied experiences of stroke victims. Each account seems as unique as the brain of the individual who wrote it. Perhaps, in the final analysis, the only way to understand what a stroke is and the lifelong impact it can bring to a patient's existence is to have sustained one and fortuitously survived with mental competencies intact. The quote from Plato at the beginning of Chapter 2 could hardly be truer.

This book was written to serve anyone interested in learning about strokes or teaching others about them. It is for a caregiver—physician, nurse, physician's assistant, physical therapist, occupational therapist, MRI technician, family member—to show the patient. It is for the patient to learn about what has happened to his brain and where the stroke has occurred. It is for students striving to learn.

We express appreciation to reviewers Susan Kaplan, associate professor, Florida International University; and Robert Sikes, associate professor, Northeastern University, for their efforts in contributing to the production of this book.

James P. Bowman
Frank D. Giddings

Chapter 1

INTRODUCTION TO STROKES AND PATIENTS

Strokes often result in extraordinary personal upheavals with lifelong consequences. They rank first as a cause of chronic and permanent functional disability. Many stroke victims recover with little or no significant consequences, but the vast
majority, as many as 3 million people in the United States, remain impaired. Stroke
also represents the third leading cause of death, after heart disease and cancer, in the
adult population in the United States. About 175,000 patients die from this cause each
year.

A commonly held belief is that there has been a gradual but steady decline in
strokes since records first became available in the early 1900s. However, it never has
been entirely clear exactly what has declined: the death (mortality) rates associated
with stroke; the incidence of stroke; or the severity of stroke. The fact is that not all
studies on any of these measures show strokes to be on the wane. Indeed, according to
a recent study, the number of strokes is rising. In 1999 alone, there were about 750,000
full-fledged strokes in the United States and some 500,000 so-called "ministrokes" or
"silent strokes" that are known medically as transient ischemic attacks (TIAs). The
problem may be even worse, however, because it is believed that ministrokes are
greatly underdiagnosed.

A ministroke results from a temporary interruption of blood flow to the brain. The
symptoms of a ministroke are usually subtle and passing. They may last anywhere
from a few seconds to a day or so and rarely cause permanent brain damage. It has
been estimated that as many as 2.5% of all adults age 18 and over have experienced
a confirmed TIA. This amounts to 4.9 million people in the United States. Furthermore, an additional 1.2 million Americans over the age of 45 may have suffered TIAs
without even realizing it.

Strokes represent the most common outcome in patients who have long-term
cerebrovascular disease. Cerebrovascular disease is a generic term referring to
any disease that affects the blood vessels of the brain. Most cerebrovascular disease can be attributed to atherosclerosis and hypertension. These two disorders are
not mutually exclusive and may interact in a variety of ways as will be explained

later. Atherosclerosis, also called arteriosclerosis, is a disease process resulting in the deposit of fat in the walls of large and medium-sized arteries. The fat deposits, called plaques, are irregularly distributed in the walls of blood vessels although they most often develop in certain favored locations. In partially occluding the passageway (the lumen) through the vessel, atherosclerotic plaques reduce the flow of blood distal to the occlusion and starve brain tissue of adequate nourishment. Atherosclerosis may also cause other vascular problems. Hypertension is a disease process resulting in chronically elevated blood pressure. This may lead to artery rupture and hemorrhage of blood into the brain. Of all cerebrovascular disorders, brain hemorrhage can be the most dramatic with the patient dying within hours.

Strokes come in all sizes and shapes but their most characteristic feature is the suddenness with which neurological signs and symptoms appear. Although this may be a matter of days in certain cases, the neurologic deficits typically develop much more rapidly than with other brain disorders, and they develop most often without an accompanying seizure. Moreover, some of the neurologic deficits usually are focal in nature, meaning that they can be attributed to an abnormality in a known and specific area of the brain. At one extreme, the onset of a stroke may be so sudden that the patient stops speaking in midsentence and simultaneously is paralyzed on one side of the body. At the other extreme, a stroke may be so mild that any neurological disability is of little or no concern to the patient and a doctor is never consulted. Thus, strokes do not always have vivid beginnings or result in significant disability.

The patient with cerebrovascular disease may experience neurological problems prior to the occurrence of an actual stroke. For example, the lumen of a blood vessel may be blocked only to the extent that there is a chronic marginal flow of blood to a specific brain area. In this circumstance, a neurologic disability, such as reduced vision, may appear only during periods of activity when the blood flow demands from other parts of the body, such as muscles, tax blood flow to the brain.

Stroke patients and their families often place difficult demands on a physician. In some cases, the particular combination of neurologic signs and symptoms enable a neurologist to locate the area of damage in the brain, sometimes so accurately that the particular arterial branch affected by the disease can be specified. However, in other cases this cannot be done and the reasons are complex. A number of factors, both structural and metabolic, specific to a particular patient may be present that make the correlation between the status of a blood vessel affected by disease and the health of the brain tissue supplied by that vessel imperfect. Especially in the case of strokes, each patient must be evaluated as an individual. For example, a blood vessel may be significantly or even completely occluded, yet the tissue supplied by that vessel may still receive an adequate supply of blood from other undamaged vessels. This means that the expected symptoms either may not appear, or their severity may be less than anticipated. A doctor simply cannot predict which of these factors might exist in a given patient, nor how the factors might interact if more than one is present. Thus, the descriptions of stroke syndromes that appear in this text are "idealized" syndromes: They present an array of deficits that *could* occur in a patient who has sustained damage to a particular blood vessel.

Beyond these biologic factors, psychological reasons exist to make the patient-physician relationship potentially difficult. The oftentimes chronic nature of neurological impairments is one of these. The mere fact that problems persist even after the patient has seen a doctor calls into question the ability of medical science to effectively treat the disorder. This places both the doctor and patient in what may be an uncomfortable position. The patient, his family, or other caregivers are frustrated because definitive advice to improve the patient's lot is not being given, and the physician may feel uncomfortable, or even helpless, in being unable to provide such information. In addition, a chronic disorder may not dominate the life of either the patient or those in his environment, including physicians, to the exclusion of all else. Life goes on. The doctor must see other patients, some with acute, perhaps life-threatening disease. Finally, it is probably unlikely that a physician has experienced chronic illness and so may lack sensitivity regarding the patient's feelings about his or her situation.

As neurological disorders go, strokes are cloaked in uncertainty. This fact makes it difficult for patients and doctors alike. After all, the unwritten contract between patient and doctor is the patient's belief that the doctor is the expert, the person in possession of the knowledge to interpret and explain the patient's condition and prospects for recovery. However, it is not always possible to even specify the cause of a stroke. The patient may feel like a victim of blind fate.

Even more uncertainty surrounds recovery. The physician is faced with a patient who has experienced a sudden event, an event seeming to have come out of nowhere, possibly at random, and an event so dramatic the patient may believe it has changed everything, perhaps forever. The patient has been profoundly altered in an instant. It is like nothing else. It is not like an evolving sickness with a known progression. It is not like going to sleep where one has the expectation that all will be the same upon waking. One minute the patient is well and the next minute the patient is sick. Patients may suddenly find themselves in a frightening world where nothing can be taken for granted: not walking, not speaking properly, not swallowing, not seeing. The patient has become a sudden prisoner in a malfunctioning body.

In the face of the brain's enormous complexity, the physician may be reduced to vague, imprecise explanations. Nerve cells fire in unknown patterns and in groups of unknown numbers, and we feel and move, think and wonder. How does a mind arise, and then think, from the physical stuff of fluids and cells? No wonder explanations are hazy and indefinite. *"We'll know better in six months how much recovery will occur." "The brain is very 'plastic' and considerable recovery sometimes occurs." "There is no cure other than time."* To the patient, and family desperately seeking definitive answers, these are not comforting, reassuring statements. But they are true.

Effective treatment of stroke victims is severely hampered by two problems. The first is that despite technological advances, our understanding of the biology of stroke remains primitive, even today. A variety of treatments await the patient upon arrival at the hospital, although at this writing none reverse brain damage that has already occurred. The second and far more important problem is simply time. Brain cells die rapidly when their blood supply is sufficiently compromised. The fact is the vast majority of people who suffer a stroke do not seek treatment until it is too late. Many people sustain strokes during sleep and are unaware of even having had one until they wake up. An average of six hours will have elapsed before a patient even gets to a hospital, and this is a few hours too late to halt the cascade of events leading to brain damage.

BLOOD SUPPLY TO THE BRAIN

The brain makes up only about 2% of total body weight (3 pounds or so), yet it consumes from 15 to 20% of the total output of blood from the heart. Why does this relatively small organ require such a large blood supply? The energy demands of brain cells, the neurons, are very high (especially during sleep!) yet they have no mechanism by which to store significant amounts of the essential nutrients that fuel their high metabolism. The essential nutrients, oxygen and glucose, are delivered to neurons by blood and thus the brain must receive a large and uninterrupted supply from the heart.

This dependence of neuron survival on a continuous and abundant blood supply is reflected in a number of facts. First, any given nerve cell is only a minute distance from a blood vessel (a capillary), no more than 20 to 50 micrometers away (Figure 1-1). Consequently, once glucose and oxygen have crossed the wall of a capillary they have to diffuse only minute distances to reach a neuron. Second, depriving the brain of its blood supply quickly results in disastrous consequences. When blood is totally prevented from reaching the brain, loss of consciousness will occur in about 10 seconds. If the brain is completely deprived of blood, nerve cells will begin to die within 3–5 minutes, causing irreversible brain damage. This is because the limited glucose and oxygen stores within neurons are exhausted in a matter of minutes and the supply of molecules the nerve cell uses to power its metabolic activity falls to zero shortly thereafter. Because of the brain's dependence on a continuous blood supply, it is not surprising to find that the brain possesses elaborate mechanisms to ensure the constancy of cerebral circulation: It is maintained by a set of reflexes under the control of centers in the lower brain stem of the central nervous system (CNS).

Two major arterial systems deliver blood to the brain. These are the internal carotid arteries and the vertebrobasilar system (Figure 1-2). The total blood flow to the brain is about 750–1000 milliliters per minute. Of this amount, about 350 ml/min flows

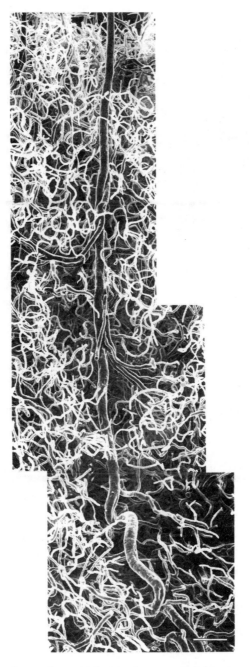

Figure 1-1. Blood vessels supplying the human cerebral cortex. The blood vessels were injected with plastic, the surrounding tissues dissolved away, and the resulting cast examined with a scanning electron microscope. The calibration bar is only 100 micrometers, which emphasizes the high density of blood vessels nourishing neurons of the cerebral cortex.
(From Duvernoy, H.M., *The Human Brain: Surface, Blood Supply, and Three-Dimensional Sectional Anatomy,* 2nd ed. New York: SpringerWien, 1999.)

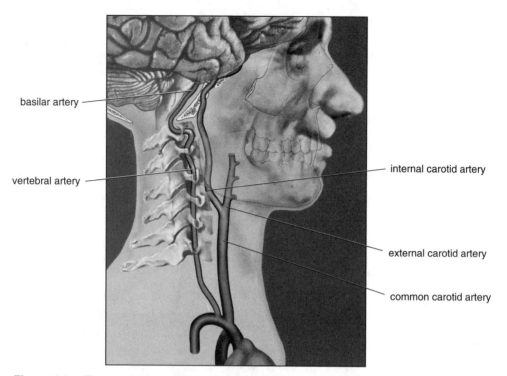

basilar artery

vertebral artery

internal carotid artery

external carotid artery

common carotid artery

Figure 1-2. The two major arterial systems that deliver blood to the brain are the internal carotid and the vertebral-basilar systems.

through each of the two carotid arteries and about 100–200 ml/min flows through the vertebrobasilar system. These normal flow differences should not be confused with the issue of importance. Both systems are vital to a normal life, they simply supply different parts of the brain. The flow differences occur because the internal carotid system supplies a larger volume of brain tissue than does the vertebrobasilar system. Strokes involving either system can be rapidly fatal or result in lifelong disabilities. After giving off a number of branches, each system reaches the base of the brain to contribute to a set of arteries called the circle of Willis. From the circle of Willis, each system gives off an elaborate network of arterial branches, each of which is named and the area of the brain supplied known. Many of these branches are common sites of stroke and will be discussed later.

THE BRAIN IS ORGANIZED IN SEEMINGLY CONTRADICTORY WAYS

The brain is organized in two seemingly contradictory ways. Both are important to our understanding of the deficits resulting from brain damage. On one hand, the organization is exceptionally precise and specific, yet at the same time, there exists a marked diffuseness in the pattern of organization. The crucial factor in this distinction is the power of the magnifying glass we select to view the brain.

If we look at single nerve cells or small collections of nerve cells (nuclei), the specificity of organization is astonishing. A single nerve cell, for example, is divisible into numerous compartments—each with specialized molecular structures for carrying out functions specific to that compartment and not shared by other compartments of the same cell. This makes one part of a nerve cell dependent upon other parts for its normal function, indeed, even its very survival. Additionally, different nerve cells may be entirely unique in terms of their biochemistry. As another example, the inputs to a single cell, and there may be thousands upon thousands originating from many other parts of the brain, are precisely located on the surface of that cell's membrane according to the specific source of the input and its importance to the function of the cell.

Collections of nerve cells within the brain gathered together in nuclei have organizations whose complexity increases with the size of the nucleus. Even small, discrete nuclei can be subdivided into distinct parts whose cells may vary in terms of their structure, biochemistry, blood supply, and connections. Regarding the connections, different cells within a nucleus receive information from different sources and project to different parts of the brain.

In areas of the brain where nerve cells are arranged in layers (the cerebral cortex, for example), one layer has functions and connections different from its immediately adjacent neighbor. Even neighboring cells in the same layer may have distinct connections and functions.

All the preceding are the structural expressions of what is known as the localization of function within the brain. What localization of function means for the stroke victim and clinical neurologist is that damage to a certain part of the brain typically results in predictable signs and symptoms different from those caused by damage to other parts of the brain.

On the other hand, if we choose to look at the fiber connections in the brain, we will be astounded to find how diffuse the connections are. One small region of the brain sends projections to many other parts of the brain, and, in turn, receives projections from many other parts. And this is the rule, not the exception. This diffuseness has even prompted researchers in brain structure to remark that it would be possible to trace a nerve impulse from one part of the brain to *any* other part over pathways of varying complexity. This interrelatedness is the structural expression of cooperation and interdependence of one part of the brain upon many other parts. It is no longer possible to regard a given part of the brain as purely "sensory" or purely "motor." What this view means for the stroke victim and clinical neurologist is that the destruction of even a localized, well-defined part of the brain will have consequences for the function of other parts.

Although apparently contradictory, these two views are, in fact, reconcilable and have two consequences for the stroke victim and neurologist. First, any damage to a specific part of the brain will result in signs and symptoms that are specifically dependent on the damaged part. The deficit is referable to that part, hence the term focal deficit. A set of focal deficits will define a syndrome. Second, and beyond this, however, any brain damage will also result in disturbances of function that were not served primarily by the damaged part, but by other parts of the brain dependent upon the damaged part for their normal function. These sometimes are referred to as "secondary," "indirect," or "associated" deficits. In some cases, they are known and predictable because the function of an undamaged area has been modified in a definite way. But in others, they are subtle, or even entirely unknown. Remaining, intact nervous tissue will adapt to the defect, and this process of adjustment in the undamaged parts will continue over time. Because of the complexity of organization of the brain, the processes of adaptation and adjustment cannot always be predicted. There is, in addition, the problem of individual variability in brain organization and function. Such subtle deficits may easily escape recognition in routine clinical examinations. Or a clinician may not even know what to look for or what to ask the patient or family, much less even have a means of showing the deficit objectively.

Unpredictability does not reflect poorly on anyone. After all, nothing changes about the way the brain is organized or functions whether we view it from either one of these two possible perspectives. There is no alteration in the structure of the brain or its function, only in our point of view.

SOME STROKE SYMPTOMS ARE ADAPTATIONS BY THE PATIENT TO COPE WITH BRAIN DAMAGE

There are a variety of symptoms of brain damage often referred to as *general* symptoms. They may include: difficulty in recalling current and past events, defects of intelligence, inappropriate or uncontrolled expressions of emotion such as anger or tearfulness, reduced ability to concentrate and pay attention, easy distractibility, increased aggression and impulsiveness, increased fatigue, reduced initiative with an unwillingness to take advantage of positive opportunities, difficulty with interpersonal relationships in which the normal motivations of others are misinterpreted, suspiciousness, avoidance of social interactions, fear of being rejected, anxiety, panic, and depression.

These deficits are not always predictable from consideration of the function(s) of the damaged part or the functions of the areas dependent on the damaged part. Such symptoms may be difficult, even impossible, for the clinician to understand and explain objectively. Yet they may be very obvious and distressing to the patient.

Depression, in reaction to having suffered a stroke with its resultant behavioral deficits, is understandable. Such reactive depression undoubtedly is present in many patients. However, more fundamentally, the depression may well have an organic basis. In some cases, the consequence of localized damage to a specific part of the brain may be to reduce the concentration of a particular neurotransmitter in the entire brain. This would upset the delicate balance normally existing between the brain's many neurotransmitters. More diffuse damage involving larger areas of the cerebral cortex could have the same outcome. Deficits in particular neurotransmitters or in the balance between transmitters are known to be implicated in depression of biologic origin (sometimes also called endogenous depression).

Besides biologic factors that contribute to a patient's signs and symptoms, it is to be understood that what we see in a stroke victim is a personality reacting to a specific set of defects. The patient's personality will actively readapt to its altered capacities and this adaptation can be another origin of a patient's signs and symptoms. The adaptation *process* is of neurological origin. However, the precise form the adaptation takes cannot be accurately predicted in advance. Here, it is essential that a careful analysis of a particular symptom be made in the context of the total situation in which it occurs. And the clinician need not be passive in this analysis, simply waiting for the symptom to reveal itself and then recording it. Symptoms that cover time frames of several hours or longer are especially difficult to assess in a clinical setting.

It is necessary for the clinician to undertake a thorough and painstaking observation of the patient's whole behavior pattern both in situations where she is able to perform successfully as well as in those in which she fails. The specific task the patient is attempting to perform may be the same in instances of success and failure: The only variable may be the context in which the performance is attempted. During a successful task performance, the patient looks animated, attentive, interested, pleased, and is cooperative. In the face of performance failure, a previously amiable patient may become evasive, sullen, irritable, or even aggressive.

There is a tendency to attribute such variation in performance to the so-called general symptoms of brain damage, that is, to variation in the patient's attention or interest, to a lack of initiative, or to abnormal fatigue or exhaustion. But this may not be the case at all. It may be that the whole behavior pattern the clinician is witnessing is caused by the patient's apprehension at being placed in a situation where a performance failure could occur. The patient may be extremely uneasy in situations where he does not know beforehand the outcome of the performance. Will a deficient performance result in severe anxiety? Will it incapacitate the patient to the extent that she cannot perform tasks she otherwise would have been able to carry out? In other words, reactions of evasiveness, irritability, etc. may be the patient's attempt to protect himself from the debilitating consequences of failure. These are the reactions of a surviving personality attempting to adjust and cope in the face of dramatically changed capacities.

THE PATIENT'S ENVIRONMENT HAS CHANGED

The ability to control our own thoughts is a product of the way our brains function. Like speaking and moving, it is an ability so basic to normal life that few of us ever think about it. With little conscious effort, we order our thoughts into understandable sequences, make sense of the constant stream of sensory information coming in from the world around us, and carry out the numerous acts of daily living with expected consequences. We function successfully in society because we have learned how to think according to a set of meanings peculiar to our culture. Our individual brains quite literally function in a community of brains. We have learned how to act and what to notice. We live in a recognizable world and experience a reality whose essential elements are common because specific mental processes exist by which the mind organizes itself for thinking and acting.

Because of the brain damage sustained by the stroke victim, however, the patient may be deprived of prior experiences and functions that enable him to react appropriately to external factors. An appropriate reaction depends, first, upon an accurate evaluation of the stimulus: What does it mean, should the stimulus be reacted to at all, what consequences could result from a particular reaction to the stimulus, etc.? The interface between the patient and his environment has changed. For the brain-damaged patient, external stimuli can acquire an exaggerated importance. The patient's performance may be determined to a much greater extent than normally by external stimuli. This may result in a distractibility that appears to an inexperienced observer to be an inability to concentrate.

From a different perspective, as adults we have expended considerable energy to create personal environments in which we are able to function effectively. A spouse is chosen, attachments formed, an occupation selected, and activities engaged in because we are able to successfully meet the demands they place upon us. If not, we change the environment (or continue to interact with it in a maladaptive way). Stated from the opposite point of view, we are not receptive to certain environmental events and so do not create a milieu in which those events routinely occur. In a very real sense, then, we have created for ourselves determinant environments.

Importantly, a patient may have an even stronger urge than a normal person to meet all demands placed upon him as well as possible. When a stroke victim continually finds himself in an environment in which he cannot meet the demands placed upon him, it is only natural that he would attempt to restrict that environment to exclude those demands. In extreme form, this protective mechanism may result in the stroke victim seeking complete self-exclusion from the world. Patients have remarked that when they are subjected to a continuous sequence of "unreasonable" demands, they have no choice but to voluntarily remain silent and completely withdraw from any social situation. Moreover, the patient may be *unaware* that his behavior is any different than prior to the stroke.

The patient's sphere of operation may become constricted in another way. Activities that previously were carried out automatically, without thought, may now require the patient's utmost attention to be carried out successfully. This may then prevent the patient from carrying out another activity at the same time. The mere effort to walk may demand such concentration that it effectively prevents other concurrent activity such as talking or admiring the beauty of the surrounding scenery.

MODELS OF DISABILITY: HOW DO HEALTH CARE PROFESSIONALS PERCEIVE THE PATIENT'S STATUS?

It is understandable that a neurologist's interest would focus on the patient's nervous system because a medical education and training in neurology have taught him or her to do just that. Neurologists have a vast catalog of information and knowledge about *a* (generic) brain in health and disease. They possess extensive and detailed knowledge about the biology of strokes. In all this education, there is a strong tendency to consider disease as though it were unrelated to the person in whom it occurs. When concepts of disease are separated from consideration of the victim, the consequences of the disease tend to be neglected or downplayed.

The patient is a unique human being, a specific person with idiosyncrasies whose capacities have been altered, sometimes fundamentally and in an instant. The patient must now function in a different world, perhaps even a profoundly different world. Changes in the patient's appearance and body and its ability to perform everyday functions may assault self-perception and the very sense of personal identity. The patient responds to the disease as a unique human being. So also do the people with whom the patient relates and upon whom he depends. How is the patient, this altered person, to be viewed? This is an especially important consideration during the patient's rehabilitation.

First, it is necessary to define the terms impairment, disability, and handicap as has been effectively done by the World Health Organization in 1980. These terms are dependent upon one another in the order just presented. *Impairment* is "any loss or abnormality of psychological, physiological, or anatomical structure or function." Impairments represent disturbances at the organ level. The organ of concern is, of course, the nervous system (brain). The impairments existing in any patient are essentially the list of deficits that have been disclosed during a conventional neurological examination. Paralysis of one leg or arm would be an example. *Disability* is "any restriction or lack (resulting from an impairment) of ability to perform an activity in the manner or within the range considered normal for a human being." Disabilities represent disturbances at the level of the person. Disabilities express themselves as something that happens in the patient's life. For example, a person who has suffered a stroke may have the *disability* of being unable to climb stairs because of the *impairment* of having a paralyzed leg. *Handicap* is "a disadvantage for a given individual, resulting from an impairment or a disability, that limits or prevents the fulfillment of a role that is normal (depending on age, sex, and social and cultural factors) for that individual." The person is at a disadvantage relative to other people so the experience of the patient is broadened again and placed in a social context. For example, the stroke victim who has the *disability* of being unable to climb stairs may suffer the *handicap* of being unable to visit his best friend who lives on the third floor of a building with no elevator.

Some health care professionals view the patient from what amounts to a physiological perspective: What functions have been lost, which have been retained, and, therefore, what is *biologically possible* for the patient to achieve in rehabilitation? In this medical model of disability, both the objectives and solutions are decided only by the professionals. Success is judged in terms of how much reduction has occurred in the patient's impairment or disability over time. How closely do the disabled person's physical and cognitive functions approach those of healthy, nondisabled persons?

However, it is clearly inappropriate to ignore the patient's desires and objectives in the process of rehabilitation. After all, it is the patient who is at the center of his or her new universe; the patient has to acquire new knowledge and skills to function as successfully as possible; the patient is subjected to demands from the environment. It may well be that patients may *want* to minimize their handicaps by addressing the underlying impairments and disabilities to reduce their severity. Patients may *want* to learn how to dress themselves without help, no matter what the amount of energy and time it requires each morning. On the other hand, other disabled patients may *not* want to exhaust themselves trying to dress independently; they may *not* want to use an hour of each morning simply dressing themselves. They would rather begin each day without feeling fatigued. In such cases, it would be more appropriate to employ someone else to dress the patient.

It is not necessary that health care professionals become experts in assessing and treating stroke victims with functional disability, only that they not ignore the patient's wishes and objectives; that they ask the patient and family members about this aspect of the illness; and that they then direct the patient to appropriate resources. Rehabilitation programs should include real-life activities and interests of the patient before the stroke occurred as well as therapy from family and friends. Rehabilitation must extend into the domestic setting because unless family and friends are given guidance and included, they too may join the patient in attempting to escape from the situation.

Chapter 2

OBSERVATIONS FROM MY OWN STROKE

It is true that the best doctors would be those who began as youths not only to learn the principles of their art but also to become familiar with as many diseased bodies as possible. It would be well if they themselves were not robust and had experienced all diseases in their own bodies.

—Plato
The Republic

I spent the evening of June 13, 1994, watching television. This was somewhat unusual for me. My wife was out of state attending professional school and a typical evening for me was spent sculpting in my studio. However, the previous evening and night I had been sick with a mild case of the flu, I thought. I had experienced several extended bouts of vomiting. At the time, I noticed I had no fever and thought that to be unusual, but paid no further attention to it. The next day, I felt recovered but passed most of the day reading. The evening of June 13 I watched several rather mindless programs, then switched channels to a special on spelunking. As several of the cavers were attempting to squeeze their way through a horribly small opening, I was gripped by such a wave of fear that I turned the television off and went to bed. "Now why did that happen?" I thought.

I woke up about 5:30 a.m. on June 14 with a raging headache, all the more notable because I almost never have headaches. I also had a mild tingling sensation on the right side of my face. I walked a bit unsteadily into my study and turned the television on. I didn't worry about being unsteady because I often am upon arising from bed. After about 30 minutes, the headache went away, and I returned to bed. I reawoke at 7 a.m. and rested for a bit while I allowed the momentary confusion of just awakening to disappear so I could orient myself to the new day. "I feel fine," I thought. But on attempting to stand I was so off balance I collapsed to the floor. I wasn't dizzy. There was no pain. I couldn't stand! I had no balance. Lying there, I realized that the tingling on the right side of my face was worse. I was having a stroke!

I crawled to the phone in the kitchen and called a colleague, "I'm having a stroke, please come and take me to the hospital." I crawled back to my bedroom, dressed while lying on the floor, then dragged myself into the living room. I managed to haul myself into a chair and was sitting there, tilted markedly to one side (unknown to me because I thought I was sitting straight up) when my friend arrived to take me to the hospital.

I was lucid and quite aware of everything going on around me. In the emergency room I was given a quick exam by the attending neurologist. When I was given the admission papers to sign, suddenly the papers, the room, the clock, the people, everything, was spinning around so wildly I couldn't do anything. My symptoms were increasing in number—a stroke in evolution. I was in the process of developing a full-blown Wallenberg syndrome.

COMMUNICATION: THE STROKE PATIENT IS UNIQUE

Like all medical specializations, clinical neurology has its own specialized vocabulary to define and describe the many signs and symptoms that may occur in a stroke patient. Professionals involved in the patient's care typically share much of this vocabulary. However, there is an unbridgeable chasm between the sick patient and healthy caregivers, family, and friends. Unless the caregiver has actually experienced a particular event, symptom, or sign, they are incapable of true understanding. A verbal description of the problem whether read from a textbook or learned from a teacher can never supplant the firsthand experience. Sympathy is necessary, even helpful, but it is not enough to attain understanding.

In my own case, one of the clearest examples involves the abnormal sensations I still experience in response to stimuli that neurologically intact people perceive as pressure or hot or cold. I experience what are known clinically as *paresthesias.* The term is defined (by Stedman's Medical Dictionary) as "an abnormal sensation, such as of burning, pricking, tickling, or tingling." The term *dysesthesia* also is used to describe these sensations. Dysesthesia is defined as "1. Impairment of sensation short of anesthesia. 2. A condition in which a disagreeable sensation is produced by ordinary stimuli." The definitions for both terms fall short as descriptions of the singular sensation I experience in response to pressure or hot or cold stimuli. The sensation is overwhelming. It involves not just a localized spot on an arm or leg where the stimulus occurs, but engulfs an entire extremity. It is not painful, but you do not want it to continue. The closest description I can give is something like the sensation experienced when a part of your body, a whole arm, for example, has been squeezed forcefully, then suddenly released.

What does it feel like to try to move an arm, leg, finger, or toe that is paralyzed? Unless you have tried, you do not know. Period. Alf Brodal, another neuroanatomist who suffered a stroke, describes this experience as follows:

> "It was a striking and repeatedly made observation that the force needed to make a severely paretic muscle contract is considerable. The expression force in this connexion refers to what one, for lack of a better expression, might call

force of innervation. Subjectively this is experienced as a kind of mental force, a power of will. In the case of a muscle just capable of being actively moved the mental effort needed is very great. Subjectively it felt as if the muscle was unwilling to contract, and as if there was a resistance which could be overcome by very strong voluntary innervation.

"This force of innervation is obviously some kind of *mental* energy which cannot be quantified or defined more closely, but the result of which is seen as a contraction of the muscle(s) in question. The expenditure of this mental energy is very exhausting, a fact of some importance in physiotherapeutic treatment. One can only speculate upon how this mental energy is ultimately transferred to mechanical energy, a question related to the apparently insoluble mind-body problem."

—Brodal, A. Self-observations and neuroanatomical considerations after a stroke. *Brain,* 1973, 96: 675–694.

Based on my own experience, I wish to expand on Brodal's comment about how he found the effort to move a paralyzed limb "very exhausting." The feeling of fatigue, sometimes overwhelming in intensity, is shared by many stroke victims. It does not relate specifically to a particular activity although it makes itself clearly known during attempts at motor activity. The underlying cause seems to be related to (or is due to) the fact that a stroke victim has to consciously direct behaviors, important components of which the undamaged brain performed automatically.

While my stroke did not cause paralysis of either arms or legs, it did damage a part of my brain stem involved with the control of balance. At first, I was unable to sit upright or stand (let alone walk) without the complete physical support of someone else. Even then I was horribly wobbly. The effort to sit upright on my own required utmost concentration. I would tip to one side and have to contract another muscle to counteract the tipping. But which muscle, which set of muscles? I did not know. Before my stroke my brain had always made this calculation for me automatically, without my having to think about it. My new brain would try to contract the correct muscles, only to miscalculate—causing me to lurch to the opposite side. Back and forth I'd go, swaying from one side to the other. Trying to figure out how to sit upright was a riveting and absolutely exhausting undertaking. I would be sweating in a matter of minutes. I remember wondering to myself "Why should I be so surprised at this?" After all, as an infant I had spent years learning about balance, about the delicate, even, and precisely timed contractions required of so many muscles in order to sit, stand, and walk. This must have required monumental effort. My brain had to learn sets of very complicated rules. But the enterprise was undertaken in a context of excitement, the excitement of newness, exploration, and adventure. The infant's brain is focused on the excitement, not the effort required and fatigue resulting from the activity. Relearning as an adult is not the same at all: It occurs in the context of having sustained a loss and having to attempt to perform tasks that previously were done effortlessly. This frustration gives fatigue a more demanding presence.

Standing and walking were even more challenging. At first, I was suspended from a stationary metal frame with a parachute harness, and held upright while my brain tried to figure out which muscles to contract to keep me standing and relatively stationary. Once I could sort of stand, I was suspended from a mobile frame on wheels and the other end of the parachute harness was strung through a pulley on the frame. One of my two physical therapists would pull on the harness to keep me upright while the other therapist, crawling along on the floor, would move my legs and feet as though I were walking. After a week of this, I was able to lurch, reel, and stagger my way down some 100 feet of hallway on my own, but it took about 30 minutes.

As a neuroanatomist, for years I had taught about the brain mechanisms involved in equilibrium and balance. I had always told students that we do not appreciate the role balance plays in everyday behavior until it has been lost. How ignorantly right I was! I truly did not understand how absolutely basic this wondrously complex act of balance is to every movement we undertake. Having to relearn this fundamental ability was unique. It was like nothing else, and it was exhausting.

In summary, what the stroke patient faces, assuming language itself has not been disrupted by the stroke, is formidable. In the first place, the patient is attempting to describe experiences that may be wholly unfamiliar to him. Such experiences are not known to the neurologically intact and had never before been experienced by the patient. Beyond this, however, the language itself is inadequate. Appropriate words simply do not exist to adequately describe the feelings, sensations, and perceptions that are occurring in the stroke victim's brain. No wonder a patient may fumble for words, or may simply give up trying to communicate altogether and passively agree with a doctor's sometimes feeble descriptions.

WHAT DOES IT MEAN TO RECOVER?

One of the understandable gulfs that exists between the stroke victim and those healthy individuals in his environment (caregivers, family, and friends) has to do with opinions about recovery. Over time, we normally experience a given person over and over again, and each such sensory experience is a separate, individual event. Another person is never experienced in her entirety at any one time. This is obvious because, for example, a friend can appear in many different circumstances and surroundings, and because during any given encounter we may pay attention to only a few of the many aspects of the context in which the person is behaving and being perceived. Physicians, in particular, typically observe the patient's behavior in the very limited, usually well-defined context of the clinic.

We look at one another, and from these observations of behavior make conclusions about the state of the person being watched. Our inevitable point of reference is ourselves, the one constant in our existence. The person is able to walk, just as *I* can; the person is able to speak, just as *I* do; and so on. From these many observations of a patient's behavior, we create a mental picture of whether the patient has recovered, and how well. But it is nothing more than a mental image, it originates in our own mind, and, unfortunately, may not accurately reflect how the patient feels about herself.

Some patients make what appear to be spectacular recoveries; they have beaten the odds, but these descriptions are likely given by other people. Stroke victims themselves have remarked that even after "all this time" when others observe that I seem to be "as I was, I am painfully aware that this is not so." I often have friends remark that I appear "fully recovered," that I appear "normal," that I have no "lingering deficits," and so on. This is not true. My stroke occurred in 1994, but to this day I have many of the deficits I initially experienced, only now they are much less intense. They are less intense perhaps because they no longer dominate my conscious awareness as they originally did, perhaps because I have learned to compensate for them, perhaps because they truly have lessened in intensity owing to structural changes in my brain. But they are there, especially when I am tired from overexertion.

Were I asked today what single factor was most important in my own recovery, it would be the capacity to pay attention to what I am doing on a moment-by-moment basis *when* I am engaged in an activity experience has shown me I will have problems with because of my stroke. I am lucky that I did not sustain a global deficit that impacts all my daily activities. For example, I have to pay attention to maintaining my balance when in an unsupported, upright position, whether standing still or moving. The slower I move, the more I have to concentrate, and the more difficulty I have. I have difficulty engaging in certain other activities at the same time, such as paying attention to scenery or wildlife while hiking. Activities that previously were "automatic," like balance in my case, have now come under "conscious cortical control." It is a compensation that has come with a price tag, namely, I am unable to do certain other things at the same time. The point here is not to list my own deficits, but to say that I remain compromised to this day. I am not fully recovered. I cannot do many of the things I did before my stroke. But if you saw me, you would say I was "normal" because you can see that I am able to walk, you can see that I am able to run, you can see that I am able to hike. You would not see that I am unable to ski.

It is quite typical for neurologists and other professionals who care for stroke patients to indicate that the process of recovery from brain damage involves two phases. The first phase is usually called the "acute" phase. It refers to the recovery that takes place during the first days, weeks, or months following the stroke. The second phase is called the "chronic" phase and it takes place during the ensuing months or years after the acute phase. The extent of brain damage, the age of the patient, and her capacities before the stroke (including cognitive status, motivation, etc.) play an important role in determining the duration of the two phases. However, it sometimes is assumed that most of the recovery following severe stroke occurs within the first six months, and that virtually all the recovery occurs during the first year or two following brain damage.

The mechanisms involved in both phases are unknown and thus speculative. The rapid and sometimes dramatic recovery during the acute phase seems likely to be a reflection of processes such as decreases in brain swelling, resorption of blood, removal of dead brain cells, alterations in cerebral blood flow and metabolism, and short-term adaptations in surviving brain cells. These are more or less global processes with widespread functional consequences and so have been speculated to account for the greatest degree of restoration of function during the overall recovery process.

The mechanisms underlying the slower and more limited recovery during the chronic phase are even more speculative. We know little about what actually takes place in the patient's brain during this stage of recovery. It has been speculated that previously inactive brain cells may become active after brain damage. This seems most unlikely. Why would there be a reserve of dormant brain cells in the first place—sets of cells just waiting for damage to occur? Why such a reserve of cells, when the damage may never come, or, if it does, arrive in an unknown place, and in an unknown way, and with an unknown intensity? And how could a dormant set of cells escape the effects of disuse atrophy ("use it or lose it")?

It would seem more likely that remaining and intact nerve cells adapt to the death of cells in other parts of the brain by altering their metabolism, growth patterns, and function in such a way that they make new connections among themselves that are able to assume some of the functions of the lost cells. But clearly the specificity of organization present in the nondamaged brain could hardly be reproduced in a damaged brain where parts have been lost. Such a process might not occur equivalently in all parts of the brain, being less satisfactory in parts of the brain possessing more complex organizations. Even if new brain cells are born during adulthood, how would the new cells know they were born into an abnormal environment requiring adjustments different from the normal pattern? The use of alternative brain regions for performing a particular task may occur, either spontaneously or with therapy.

As noted, the chronic phase sometimes is considered to have a limited life span, in the neighborhood of several years, so that little, if any, additional recovery can be expected to occur after this cut-off point. This seems to be an unduly pessimistic assumption about recovery. The relatives of patients with brain damage often report gradual and steady improvement over periods as long as 14 or 15 years. Recent studies with patients sustaining traumatic brain injury report significant improvements in cognitive functions, motor functioning, behavioral response to the environment, initiative-independence, and social and interpersonal functioning for at least 10 years post-injury. One such study concludes:

> "Our findings suggest that clinicians working with patients who sustain severe traumatic brain injury should refrain from telling the brain-injured patients and/or their family or significant others that most or all of the recovery

should occur within 1–2 years post-injury. Sbordone [5] has pointed out that such feedback only serves to exacerbate the brain-injured patient's depression, and creates a loss of hope, which reinforces the patient's depression and feelings of frustration. With this in mind, it should be recognized that the dictum 'Do no harm,' which is part of the Hippocratic oath taken by every physician, should be heeded and practiced by professionals who work with brain injured patients."

—From Sbordone, R.J. et al. Recovery of function following severe traumatic brain injury: a retrospective 10-year follow-up. *Brain Injury,* 1995, 9: 285–299.

THOUGHTS ABOUT DYING . . . AND LIVING

We are unable to comprehend much that exists in our world, whatever the reason may be, say, lack of appropriate training or thought patterns that do not allow understanding. But what I speak of here is an element of life that reason and intellect alone do not prepare us to comprehend, even remotely. There is a vital realm of experience, beyond love and empathy, that gives rise to understanding. It is a door that had remained closed to me before my stroke. Indeed, I had not even realized the door existed, until it opened.

Yet here I was standing at the threshold, preparing to enter a dark room to experience something wholly unfamiliar. In my search for understanding and meaning in my life, had I been like a flashlight? Asked to find something in this dark room that did not have light shining upon it, my flashlight-self would have to conclude that there is light on everything, since there was light in whatever direction I turned.

Before my stroke, my perception of my world had been clouded by the verbal notions in which I did my thinking. I was taught to think and experience in this verbal way. My formal education seemed to have failed to accomplish one of the important things it was supposed to do: Help me understand the nonhuman otherness of the world. I had, as it were, been petrified by language, flopping about in a world of reduced awareness. It occurred to me that Western scientific thought was very limiting. Limiting because it teaches us to believe that all questions, even the cosmic ones like meaning and purpose, can be dissected and understood if only we ask the right questions. An inability to understand stems from our being unable to frame the right questions, to reduce things to their most fundamental components: All can be known, if only we know how to ask. But in the back of my mind was the thought that wiser cultures know otherwise: Alternative states of consciousness allow the experiencing of other realities.

If the doors of perception were cleansed everything would appear to man as it is, infinite.

For man has closed himself up, till he sees all things thro'
narrow chinks of his cavern.

—William Blake, from *The Marriage of Heaven and Hell,* 1790–1793

The door opened during the period of time my stroke was evolving and the symptoms worsening. My training gave me the knowledge that the first 36 or so hours were ones in which I was indeed floating about in a world of total uncertainty. At the time, I knew the brain area in which my stroke had occurred was critical, near vital centers in the brain stem controlling respiration, heart rate, and blood pressure. I lay in intensive care thinking and feeling. I did not sleep for those 36 hours. I wanted to know, clearly and exactly, how I was changing. I was not afraid of the unknown, I was not afraid of dying. Here I had spent much of my life trying to find ways to prolong my life expectancy, only to come to the understanding that dying is not something I feared. It must be a mental state we enter when we instinctively know that all is utterly, completely, totally beyond our control.

This singular condition was not the result of any mental process I had chosen. It was something that just happened. I was quite conscious of all the goings on in my environment: A new symptom would appear, another recede to the background, waxing and waning as they wove themselves through my awareness; family and friends would arrive and leave; doctors and nurses would arrive, poke and prod, scratch, and tap doing their various neurological tests. My situation had simply annihilated any fear of death.

I knew things never could return to the way they were. My understanding of what it means to be alive had changed. But what about the predicament of living life as a handicapped person? Would I have to adapt my life to some seemingly hopeless situation? Would I be facing a lifetime of restricted activities, of missed opportunities? Would I experience feelings of inferiority and self-consciousness? I thought of a scene I witnessed many years ago. A crippled lady crossing a busy street corner. The act seemed to require superhuman strength as she resolutely forced one foot before the other in front of the idling cars stopped temporarily by the red light. Some drivers looked impatient as her twisted body moved slowly ahead. Would she get across before the traffic light turned green? The expressions on the drivers' faces betrayed a mixture of pity, disgust, and curiosity. The traffic light changed before she had crossed all the way. Fortunately, only a single horn honked. But that sorrowful horn caused her face to break into a smile as she continued her struggle. I remember wondering why she smiled. What did she know? Perhaps I now understand. Nothing in the world need be changed even if the way I experience it may be different.

DOES A STROKE ADD ANYTHING TO ONE'S LIFE?

There is, of course, no definitive or uniform answer to the question of whether a stroke adds anything to the victim's life. This depends on the severity of the stroke, the areas of the brain affected, the extent of recovery, and the patient's thought processes and concerns before the stroke. But certainly it is not an uncommon re-action for patients to indicate that a stroke paradoxically improved the quality of their lives (provided the stroke did not impair their mental capacities). In some cases, disease may even inspire its victim to seek new insights into the human con-dition. This clearly was the case with John Donne, the English divine and poet of the late sixteenth and early seventeenth centuries, who wrote extensively about his spiritual quest inspired by a struggle with sickness. The deep insights Donne gained from this search appear in his book *Devotions Upon Emergent Occasions.* Donne is, perhaps, most familiar to us for a specific writing in his Seventeenth Meditation:

> *"Any Mans* death *diminishes* me, *because I am involved in* Mankinde*;*
> *And therefore never send to know for whom the* bell *tolls;*
> *It tolls for* thee . . .*"*

After my stroke, I became acutely aware that I had been making two simulta-neous journeys through life. One was outside of myself, it took place in my social environment as a result of my own actions and the actions and opinions of others. The other journey was within myself, a journey of thoughts and dreams where I could imagine myself doing things I was not actually doing, and with imagined out-comes and consequences. This internal journey would sometimes collide with the facts of my outside journey as when, of my own free will, I would do something that met with disagreement from others in my life. Before my stroke, the collision could easily prompt me to conclude that there was something amiss about my internal journey, that my thought was wrong and needed tweaking, or that my dream was un-attainable. But after my stroke, I felt strangely disconnected, distanced from my ex-ternal journey. Sometimes I wondered whether I was even still on an external journey, whether its importance had disappeared altogether. Of course I still am on that external journey, but its importance is less, the sting of negative reactions has been diminished.

I learned to value highly the capacities I relearned after my stroke as well as those I retained, and stand in awe of their enormous complexity. I think of the patience of parents and others who kindly spend so many years mentoring us as infants and chil-dren as we gradually learn these complex skills. Postural stability, walking, swallow-ing, seeing, gazing steadily at an object, speaking, and thinking are not the hardy and stable elements of everyday life they seem to be, but fragile and extraordinary capac-ities that can be ripped away in an instant.

> *"Love your eyes that can see, your mind that can*
> *Hear the music, the thunder of the wings. Love the wild swan."*

—Robinson Jeffers, from *Love the Wild Swan,* 1935

My awareness of the many elements ongoing in my life has expanded tremendously: My wife and family; the smell of the Pacific Ocean and the rhythm of its pounding surf; flickering flames wandering over the surface of fireplace logs; the glow of molten bronze cascading into a mold; our dog quietly going about its business of being a little animal; the red-yellow flare that brilliantly colors the eastern sunrise. . . . Each of these occupies a greater volume in my mind. Sometimes it is as though the very act of perceiving something swallows up its concept. I am luckier than most, no doubt. No doubt.

Chapter 3

GENERAL INFORMATION ABOUT STROKES

THE STROKE SYNDROME

The most important feature of a stroke is the time course over which behavioral deficits unfold. Most typically, the functional disability develops rapidly and this distinguishes a stroke from other brain disorders, such as tumors, which develop more slowly. The patient may awaken and be unable to get out of bed or to speak. A patient may be suddenly paralyzed and fall to the ground. When the neurologic deficit does not reach a peak almost at once, it may evolve in a series of steps over a period of minutes, hours, and sometimes days. Each step is characterized by the appearance of a new deficit or set of deficits.

Most stroke victims then experience a stabilization of their deficits. Again, this occurs rather quickly, over a matter of a day or so. This rapid stabilization distinguishes stroke from progressive neurological disorders in which there is a steady or step-wise deterioration of function.

Recovery of function then begins. This may occur quite suddenly or over weeks or months. Contrary to much current opinion, the recovery process may continue for years although at a slower pace than originally. With small strokes, residual disabilities may be minimal or even nonexistent. However, patients suffering more severe (larger) strokes may be left with considerable functional impairment, sometimes for the remainder of their lives.

In sum, the hallmark of a stroke is its temporal profile: short relative to other diseases of the brain. And this limited time frame may apply to all aspects of the disorder: its onset and the development of deficits; the attainment of stabilization; and the resolution of the deficits. Note that we have said nothing here about the cause of a stroke.

TYPES OF CEREBROVASCULAR DISEASE

Most cerebrovascular disease falls into one of two categories: either ischemic or hemorrhagic. Ischemic stroke is by far the most common and accounts for about 80 percent of all stroke. The term ischemia means to *keep back blood*. Ischemia is due to mechanical obstruction of one or more arteries so that blood distal to the site of the occlusion is reduced to a level inadequate to sustain normal neuronal activity. Whether or not ischemia results in cell death depends on its severity and duration. When ischemia is severe, neurons and other cells in brain tissue deprived of blood soon die and this is called ischemic necrosis, the term *necrosis* meaning *to make dead*. The local area of necrotic brain tissue is referred to as an infarct. Infarcts due to ischemia often result in what are called pale infarcts because there are no red blood cells in the area of the infarct. The infarcted tissue therefore is pale in appearance. This type of stroke generally affects the older population.

With hemorrhagic disorders, arteries rupture and blood floods from the broken vessel directly into brain tissue, into the ventricles of the brain, or into the small space surrounding the brain (the subarachnoid space). The infarct is then referred to as a red or hemorrhagic infarct due to the presence of red blood cells in the affected tissue. This type of stroke may affect both younger and older people.

Intracranial hemorrhage has two major effects on brain tissue. The first is because the volume of blood that has escaped from an artery takes up space inside the skull (within the cranial vault). This space normally is occupied by brain cells and their associated fluids, but in the face of the space-occupying hemorrhage, brain cells must give way to accommodate this new volume of fluid. The problem is that in an adult, the bony cranial vault will not expand to accommodate this increased volume. This can result in a number of problems. For one thing, it may cause a rise in intracranial pressure, which then automatically reduces blood flow into the brain resulting in local or whole-brain ischemia. Of more immediate concern is that the mass of blood may be sufficiently large to compress brain tissue. Such compression can cause direct tissue destruction, or it can cause other arteries themselves to be compressed to the point of narrowing or shutting down completely. Finally, when sufficiently large, the volume of escaped blood may cause such a rise in intracranial pressure that brain tissue itself is displaced from its normal location inside the cranial vault. This is the process of brain herniation. It can have dire consequences as the herniated brain tissue may compress parts of the brain vital to the patient's very survival.

The second major effect of intracranial hemorrhage is caused when the escaped blood irritates structures adjacent to the hemorrhage. For example, hemorrhage into the subarachnoid space causes cerebral vasospasm. In cerebral vasospasm there is a reduction in the diameter of large intracranial arteries that can persist for weeks. The resulting ischemia can be severe enough to cause further infarction.

Causes of focal cerebral ischemia vary widely, but the end result in brain tissue is the same, namely, lack of an adequate blood supply. Occlusive cerebrovascular disorders resulting in ischemia are caused primarily by atherosclerosis of blood vessels coupled with thrombosis, both leading to narrowing of the vessel lumen (Figure 3-1A). Cerebral embolism is also a cause of ischemia and is due to an embolus, usually from sources outside the brain. Inflammation of blood vessels and blood disorders may also lead to ischemia.

A

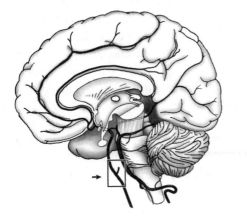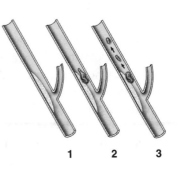

B

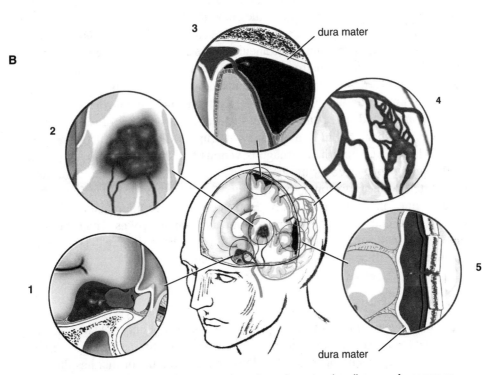

dura mater

dura mater

Figure 3-1. The two major categories of cerebrovascular disease. A, common causes of ischemic disorders: 1, atherosclerosis; 2, thrombosis; 3, embolism. B, common causes of hemorrhagic disorders: 1, ruptured aneurysm and subarachnoid hemorrhage; 2, primary intracerebral hemorrhage; 3, subdural hemorrhage; 4, ruptured arteriovenous malformation; 5, epidural hemorrhage. Subdural hemorrhage and epidural hemorrhage usually are a result of trauma to the head and, therefore, are not classified as strokes.

Atherosclerosis causes the deposition of fatty material in the walls of large- and medium-sized arteries in either their extracranial or intracranial portions (Figure 3-1A,1). The depositions of fatty material are called atherosclerotic plaques. Although atherosclerosis narrows the lumen of a vessel, it usually is not severe enough by itself to result in tissue infarction. Complete occlusion of a vessel by atherosclerosis is almost unknown.

Complete occlusion of a brain artery is due to a thrombus superimposed on an atherosclerotic plaque (Figure 3-1A,2). By causing changes in the way blood flows through the narrowed vessel, atherosclerotic plaques represent sites at which a thrombus can develop. A thrombus is a "clot" formed from cells and chemicals that are normally circulating in the blood. Attached to the vessel wall, a thrombus may completely or incompletely occlude the lumen of a vessel. The term *thrombosis* refers to the formation or presence of a thrombus.

An embolus is a plug composed of a detached fragment of a thrombus, a detached fragment of atheromatous material, or other foreign body (Figure 3-1A,3). An embolus will travel freely in the arterial circulation until it lodges in an artery whose lumen is too small to allow further passage of the embolus. This process is called embolism.

Hemorrhagic cerebrovascular disorders are caused by chronic high blood pressure (hypertension); by the rupture of aneurysms resulting from congenital factors or infection; by arteriovenous malformations; or by trauma.

Primary intracerebral hemorrhage is caused by the direct leakage of blood from an artery into brain tissue (Figure 3-1B,2). Subarachnoid hemorrhage is bleeding into the subarachnoid space surrounding the brain and spinal cord. The most common cause of subarachnoid hemorrhage is a ruptured saccular (berry) aneurysm (Figure 3-1B,1). Subdural hemorrhage is venous bleeding into the potential space beneath the dura mater covering the brain (Figure 3-1B,3) while epidural hemorrhage is arterial bleeding from a torn meningeal artery with the blood accumulating outside the dura mater (Figure 3-1B,5). Both subdural and epidural hemorrhage usually are due to head trauma and then are not classified as strokes. The rupture of an arteriovenous malformation also leads to brain hemorrhage (Figure 3-1B,4). Each of these processes will be discussed in more detail later.

RISK FACTORS

Because effective treatment of stroke patients usually is not undertaken soon enough after a stroke to prevent brain damage, it is important to eliminate as many risk factors from the person's life as possible. Unfortunately, the factor that has the highest correlation with increased stroke incidence is simply age: The passage of time allows chronic risk factors to exert a progressively increasing effect.

After age, cardiac disease is the largest risk factor for stroke. Atrial fibrillation (AF) is a common heart disease and patients often are unaware of having this condition. AF is by far the main cause of cardiac embolism. In AF there is no effective atrial contraction, which leads to stagnation of blood in the atrium of the heart. Stagnation is the major factor causing thrombosis. The sudden onset of AF or of return to a normal atrial contraction from AF causes a fragment of the thrombus to embolize. Most emboli are small and are stopped in medium-sized arteries such as the middle cerebral artery or its branches, especially on the left side of the brain. However, myocardial infarction, endocarditis, mitral valve prolapse, and other heart conditions can lead to cardiac embolism.

Hypertension is a risk factor. For one thing, hypertension worsens the process of atherosclerosis, seemingly by "driving" it into the walls of smaller diameter arteries. Further, hypertension is a specific causative factor in primary intracerebral hemorrhage, with as many as 90% of patients with this type of stroke having a history of hypertension. Hypertension is the most modifiable of the major risk factors.

Stress is one of those words that common usage (in modern Western society at least) has almost defined out of existence. Often we hear someone say how "stressed out" they are over some event that is a normal demand of their everyday life situation, say, a student who has an upcoming exam, or a self-employed accountant facing the approaching deluge of clients at income tax time. In terms of our present consideration, the only element such usage does correctly capture is that the person is referring to an external event, an environmental situation they must face. Where the usage becomes incorrect is that the "stressed out" person, in fact, has control over his response to the event: The student either prepares adequately for the exam or does not; the accountant either accepts a manageable number of clients and schedules them appropriately or does not.

It is true, of course, that there is a normal stress to which we are all are occasionally subject, a stress that is provoked by adverse life circumstances. As a reaction to the normal disappointments and occurrences of everyday life, we all experience feelings of resentment, unhappiness, discouragement, self-doubt, and an inability to control events or situations. Such normal feelings are closely related in their duration to the events that triggered them. Unfortunately, such stress has become an increasingly pervasive feature of modern life.

The essential ingredients that make an external event stressful and a risk factor in the development of disease are that the challenge is of such duration and intensity as to overwhelm the person's ability to cope with the challenge—the person has lost control and can see no end to the situation. For example, individuals forced to work under constant danger and in confined conditions, cultural groups uprooted from their homes and forced to abandon their traditional ways of life, and people subjected to repeated physical and mental abuse lose their coping skills.

Stress elicits a wide variety of normal body responses. These vary in intensity and quality depending importantly on the duration of the environmental stressor. The purpose of such normal biological reactions is to enable the person to deal effectively with the stress until it has passed. But when the stress extends over a prolonged period of time and the person perceives no end to it, a sustained version of a usually temporary set of body reactions results. This is a problem because the body is being bombarded by a continued onslaught of hormones designed to be present over limited periods of time and at extremely low levels.

It has been accepted for years that the risk factors for stroke are in general the same as those for coronary heart disease. The process of atherosclerosis in brain arteries is identical to that in the aorta, heart, and other large peripheral arteries. It runs a parallel course in both peripheral and brain arteries, although it may be somewhat less severe in the latter. Stress has long been accepted as a risk factor in the development of coronary heart disease. A recent study has confirmed that stress is a major risk factor for stroke as well.

Diabetes mellitus is a risk factor because the disease accelerates the rate of atherosclerosis. Accelerated atherosclerosis occurs in both large and small arteries.

Blood lipids are associated with increased risk of stroke in various ways. Elevated cholesterol *per se* is an uncertain risk factor for stroke and exerts its greatest threat to health by affecting the heart and peripheral blood vessels. People with low blood levels of high-density lipoprotein (HDL) and high blood levels of low-density lipoprotein (LDL) are at greater risk of developing coronary artery occlusion and cerebral atherosclerosis than people with the reverse HDL-LDL ratio. High-density lipoprotein picks up cholesterol from tissue cells and transports it to the liver for disposal. Therefore, HDLs help prevent atherosclerosis (that is, they are antiatherogenic).

Smoking (cigarettes in particular) increases the risk of stroke to a degree depending on the person's smoking habit. Even light smoking (less than one pack per day) doubles the risk of stroke. Cessation of smoking significantly reduces this risk such that five years after quitting the risk is the same as in age-matched controls who never smoked. Long-duration smoking appears to decrease HDL cholesterol and reduces cerebral blood flow.

Alcohol consumption affects stroke risk to a degree dependent upon the level of intake. Light to moderate consumption reduces the incidence of coronary artery disease, but the effect on stroke is less clear. Heavy alcohol consumption is associated with increased risk of cerebral hemorrhage because it promotes hypertension, elevated lipid blood levels, and weight gain.

The regular use of oral contraceptives increase the risk of stroke, especially in women who have increasing headaches and who smoke cigarettes. Young women normally have a very low incidence of stroke. The risk is correlated with the dose of estrogens and is particularly increased in women over 35.

Stroke incidence varies considerably between different races. Chinese, Japanese, and African-Americans have a high incidence of vascular occlusive disease and cerebral hemorrhage.

THE RELATIONSHIP BETWEEN VESSEL OCCLUSION AND CLINICAL DEFICITS CANNOT ALWAYS BE PREDICTED ACCURATELY

The actual effect of arterial occlusion on brain tissue depends on a number of factors specific to each patient. Therefore, there is not a one-to-one relationship between arterial occlusion and the state of the brain tissue supplied by the occluded vessel. As a result, the clinical deficits present in a patient cannot always be accurately predicted even when the occluded vessel is known. Much of this unpredictability stems from individual differences in structural or vascular architecture. Other factors are systemic in nature and relate to the individual's overall body and brain metabolism.

First, the structure of the circle of Willis may vary considerably in different patients (Figure 3-2). The circle of Willis is the ring of arteries at the base of the brain where the internal carotid and vertebrobasilar systems form anastomotic links. The circle is fully intact with all its pieces of significant size in only 50 percent of people. In some individuals, the structure may be such as to enable the circle of Willis to provide effective collateral circulation when there is occlusion of one internal carotid artery in the neck. This would permit the intracranial arteries on the occluded side to be filled from the opposite, unoccluded internal carotid artery thereby preventing or reducing the severity of brain infarction. In other individuals, the posterior cerebral artery of one side may arise from the internal carotid artery rather than from the basilar artery as it usually does (Figure 3-2B,2). In such cases, occlusion of the internal carotid artery on that side would result not only in the classic symptoms of carotid occlusion but also symptoms associated with occlusion of the posterior cerebral artery, making the resulting neurological deficits more extensive.

Second, natural communications, called anastomoses, occur between cerebral blood vessels (Figure 3-3). These anastomoses unite, end-to-end, branches of the three major cerebral arteries. They occur within the sulci of each hemisphere and are not visible on the surface of the adult brain. They are referred to as meningeal anastomoses and they occur in the border zones of the territories of each artery (Figure 3-4A). There are many individual variations in the number and size of these anastomotic channels. In some individuals, when there is occlusion of one of the major arteries, these interarterial anastomoses may be sufficiently robust to carry enough blood into the compromised territory to lessen the degree of ischemic infarction (Figure 3-4B). But only rarely are the end-to-end anastomotic channels large enough to support instant retrograde blood flow from one territory to another sufficient to prevent some ischemic damage. In other individuals, the anastomoses may be insufficient to prevent ischemia from occurring over the entire vascular territory of the occluded vessel.

Third, anastomoses between the internal and external carotid arteries occur to a variable degree in different individuals. One region in which such anastomoses occur is around the orbit of the eye with blood passing from the external carotid into the internal carotid artery via the ophthalmic artery (Figure 3-5). Such anastomoses may serve to lessen ischemic damage when the internal carotid artery is occluded.

Fourth, general systemic and metabolic factors may affect the degree of ischemia resulting from occlusion of a vessel. Blood pressure is one such factor.

A

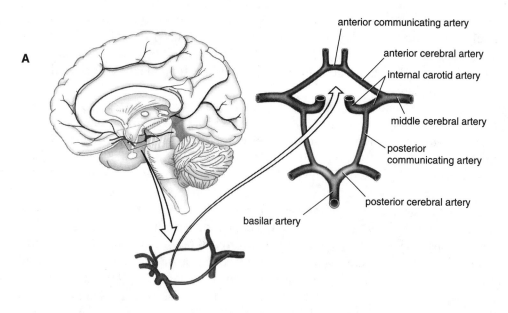

anterior communicating artery

anterior cerebral artery

internal carotid artery

middle cerebral artery

posterior communicating artery

posterior cerebral artery

basilar artery

B

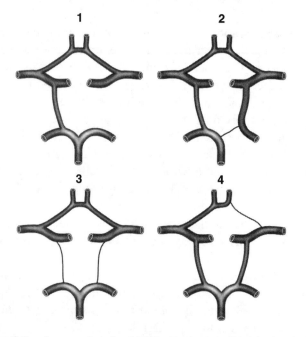

Figure 3-2.   A, normal circle of Willis. B, abnormalities in the circle of Willis: 1, incomplete circle; 2, one posterior cerebral artery arising from an internal carotid artery; 3, abnormally small posterior communicating arteries; 4, both anterior cerebral arteries perfused primarily by one internal carotid artery.

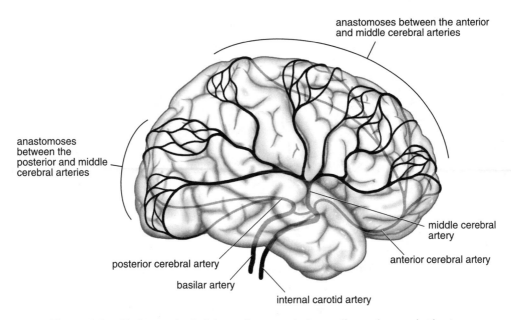

Figure 3-3.   End-to-end arterial anastomoses between the major cerebral arteries. The right cerebral hemisphere is shown. These anastomoses lie within the sulci of the cerebrum and are not visible on the surface of the adult brain. The extent and size of these anastomoses influence the potential severity of an infarct resulting from a blockage of just one of the arteries participating in the anastomosis.

Thus, a narrowed vessel may still deliver sufficient blood when blood pressure is 190/100 but fail to do so when blood pressure falls to 120/70. Such a drop in blood pressure may occur on sudden standing after a long period of recumbancy, during sleep, or in a patient who is being treated with medication designed to lower blood pressure. Likewise, a narrowed vessel may deliver sufficient blood when metabolic conditions are normal but fail to do so when metabolic conditions change. A fall in the level of sodium in blood serum; development of a fever; changes in the level of oxygen in the blood, as in patients with pulmonary disease; and lowered blood glucose levels, as in diabetics using insulin; all may result in the appearance of focal neurologic symptoms.

Fifth, the speed of occlusion may affect the ischemic outcome. When an occlusion develops slowly, more time is allowed for collateral circulation to open up. However, even though the size of functioning collateral channels increases with time, this usually occurs far too late to reduce the original risk of ischemia and infarction. Thus, when robust collateralizations are observed on angiograms performed long after strokes have been completed this does not reflect conditions at the time of the stroke. It likely is that the robust collateralization is simply perfusing the healed scars of infarction.

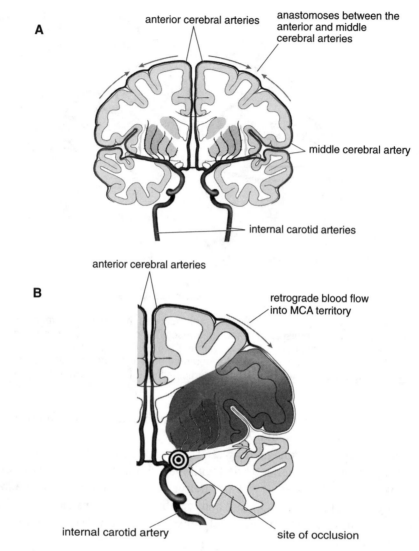

A

anterior cerebral arteries

anastomoses between the anterior and middle cerebral arteries

middle cerebral artery

internal carotid arteries

anterior cerebral arteries

B

retrograde blood flow into MCA territory

internal carotid artery

site of occlusion

Figure 3-4.   Coronal sections through the front of the brain with the anterior portions of the frontal and temporal lobes removed. The major vessels of the internal carotid system are shown. Arteries of the vertebro-basilar system are not illustrated. A, the arrows indicate one of the sites where, at each systole of the heartbeat, blood flows meet at a "dead point" in potential collateral channels formed by end-to-end arterial anastomoses between the middle and anterior cerebral arteries. B, an occlusion is shown near the origin of the middle cerebral artery (MCA). The territory supplied by the penetrating branches of the MCA (the lenticulostriate arteries) will be infarcted, as indicated by the dark shading. However, the extent of the infarct in the territory of the cortical branches of the MCA depends on the capacity of the meningeal anastomoses with the unoccluded anterior cerebral artery for retrograde (collateral) flow, as shown by the arrow and light shading. Branches of the inferior division of the MCA are not shown.

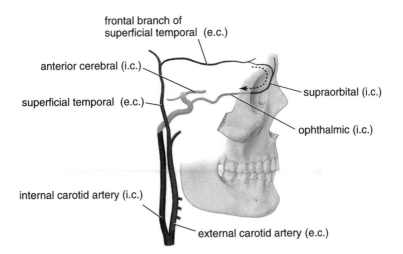

Figure 3-5. Anastomoses between the internal and external carotid arteries around the orbit of the eye via the ophthalmic artery. The extent of these anastomoses may modify the severity of cerebral ischemia. Abbreviations: e.c., external carotid; i.c., internal carotid.

Chapter 4

ATHEROTHROMBOTIC INFARCTION

THE ORIGIN OF ATHEROSCLEROSIS

The process of atherosclerosis is the same in brain arteries as it is in arteries of other parts of the body, for example, the aorta and coronary arteries. In most cases, atherosclerosis is a progressive disease. The disease has its onset in childhood and adolescence. Atherosclerotic deposits then develop and enlarge silently for 20 to 30 or more years before causing a stroke and neurologic problems.

There are two prominent theories on the origin of atherosclerosis. One is called the injury-healing hypothesis (Figure 4-1). The injury-healing hypothesis states that the initial event in the development of atherosclerosis is an inflammatory response to some factor that injures the endothelial cells making up the wall of the blood vessel. The injury could be mechanical, such as hypertension, or it could be due to increased levels of low-density lipoprotein (LDL) in the blood. The various types of cells that participate in the initial inflammatory response to injury then liberate chemicals called growth factors, which in time cause the development of atherosclerotic plaques.

The second hypothesis is called the lipid hypothesis. The lipid hypothesis asserts that excess cholesterol in blood serum initiates atherosclerosis by accumulating in blood vessel endothelial cells. Excess cholesterol is derived either from the synthesis of cholesterol by the liver or from dietary sources, or both. The accumulation may be due to a failure in what is called reverse cholesterol transport. The term reverse cholesterol transport refers to the mechanisms by which cholesterol is delivered *from* peripheral cells, including the vascular endothelial cells, *to* the liver for disposal, primarily as bile. High-density lipoproteins (HDLs) are involved in transporting cholesterol *from* peripheral cells and donating it to the liver for bile formation. Low-density lipoproteins (LDLs), on the other hand, deliver cholesterol *to* body cells. Thus, individuals with low levels of HDL and high levels of LDLs are especially prone to develop cerebral atherosclerosis. This is because of a deficiency in the mechanism that delivers cholesterol to the liver for disposal, along with an increase in the mechanism

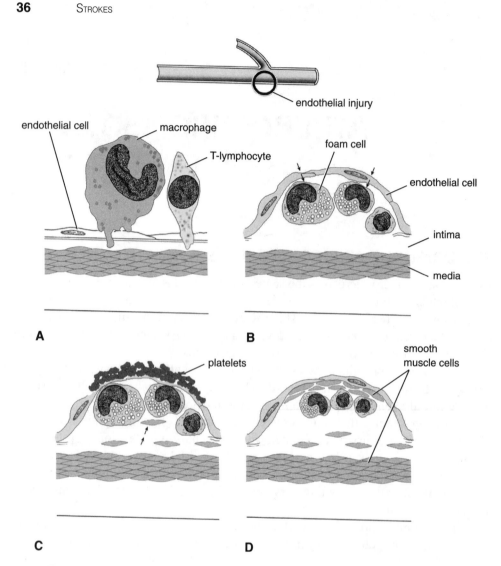

Figure 4-1. The arterial lesion in atherosclerosis according to the injury-healing hypothesis. Injury to the endothelial cells making up the wall of the artery permits circulating mononuclear cells to attach to the vessel wall (A). They then migrate beneath the endothelial layer (B) where they transform into foam cells and form a fatty streak. Blood platelets then attach to the fatty streak (C) and smooth muscle cells proliferate (D) to form the fibrous plaque characteristic of atherosclerosis. The plaque partially occludes the lumen of the artery and may cause a variety of other problems.

that delivers cholesterol to body cells like those making up the walls of blood vessels.

Atherosclerotic plaques form most easily on arterial surfaces where blood flow direction changes (Figure 4-2). Such flow changes occur at points where arteries bifurcate or where they curve sharply. The most common site in the carotid system is where the common carotid artery bifurcates into the internal and external carotid ar-

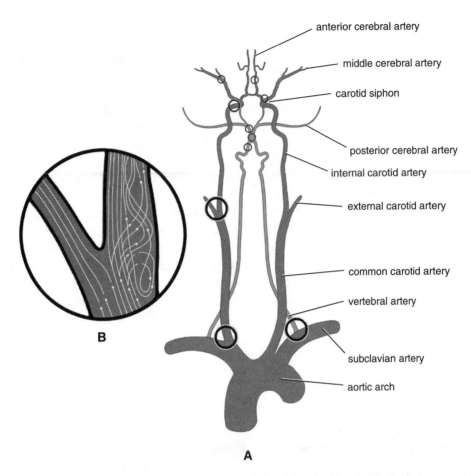

Figure 4-2. A, major sites of atherosclerosis involving the blood vessels that supply the brain. B, distortions in the laminar pattern of blood flow occur at points where blood vessels bifurcate or branch. The swirling motion of blood flow favors the development of atherosclerosis at these sites.

teries. Atherosclerosis develops at the origin of the internal carotid (in the neck) or in the first few centimeters of the internal carotid artery after its origin. The next most common site is in the carotid siphon, located just after the internal carotid artery enters the skull where the artery curves sharply. In the vertebrobasilar system, atherosclerosis most commonly occurs at the origin of the vertebral arteries in the neck, in the distal portion of the vertebral artery inside the cranium, and in the basilar artery.

There must be at least a 70 percent reduction in the diameter of a vessel before arterial pressure distal to the occlusion drops to the point where tissue nourishment is insufficient. *Stenosis* is the term used to refer to a narrowing of the vessel lumen. Cerebral atherosclerosis this severe is unusual so that atherosclerosis alone does not usually cause ischemia and infarction. As noted earlier and discussed next, in order to narrow the lumen of an artery enough to cause ischemia and infarction it is usually necessary for a thrombus to form on top of an existing atherosclerotic plaque.

The complications associated with atherosclerosis are what most often lead to neurologic signs and symptoms. These are shown in Figure 4-3. For one thing, an atherosclerotic plaque changes the surface of the vessel wall such that there is a stagnation (stasis) of blood immediately distal to the plaque. The plaque may also cause the vessel wall itself to ulcerate. Stasis and ulceration both may result in the formation of a thrombus at the site of the plaque (Figure 4-3B) The process of thrombosis then produces additional stenosis that may lead to severe and even complete occlusion of the vessel. In general, the more severe the atherosclerosis, the more likely it is that there will be thrombosis. Furthermore, fragments of the thrombus may break off and travel as emboli into the distal circulation (Figure 4-3C) Finally, ulceration of the vessel wall at the site of an atherosclerotic plaque may also lead to fragments of atheromatous material such as cholesterol breaking off and traveling as emboli (Figure 4-3D).

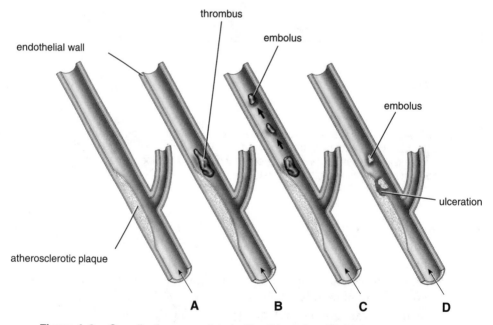

Figure 4-3.   Complications associated with atherosclerosis. A, plaque encroaching on the lumen of an artery leading to stagnation of blood flow distal to the plaque. B, formation of a thrombus on the plaque. C, fragments of the thrombus breaking off from the main mass to form emboli. D, ulceration of the vessel wall allowing material of the atherosclerotic plaque to embolize.

In many cases, stenosis of a vessel may result only in episodes of transient signs and symptoms and not produce actual tissue destruction. These transient episodes due to vascular insufficiency are called transient ischemic attacks (TIAs). Most TIAs last from 2 to 15 minutes, and rarely over 30 minutes. TIAs are a strong predictor of an impending major stroke with cerebral infarction. A stroke may follow one or more TIAs by hours, weeks, or months.

The symptoms associated with TIAs are variable and may include:

- Severe headache with no apparent cause.
- Numbness, tingling, or weakness in the face, arm, or leg, especially on only one side of the body.
- Difficulty walking.
- Difficulty talking or understanding what others are saying.
- Confusion.
- Difficulty with vision in one or both eyes.
- Dizziness and loss of coordination.

CLINICAL COURSE AND PROGNOSIS

Two stages can be identified in atherothrombotic strokes because of the length of time required for significant thrombosis to develop. The first stage is known as stroke in evolution and may last a matter of hours or a day or longer. This is the stage during which impairment of function increases in severity with time. The stage of completed stroke refers to a sustained ischemic event resulting in neurologic deficits that can last days, weeks, or permanently. It should be noted that a patient who has suffered one thrombotic stroke is at risk of having another stroke at the same or a different site in the months or years following the first stroke.

The onset of a thrombotic stroke may occur in several ways. Most often a thrombotic stroke occurs during sleep. The patient awakens unaware that he is paralyzed and falls to the floor when attempting to arise and walk. There may be only a single attack and the full stroke then evolves in a matter of hours. Alternatively, symptoms may appear in a stepwise fashion over a period of several hours or a day or two. Such intermittent progression is of particular help in diagnosing the occurrence of thrombotic stroke.

The course of an atherothrombotic stroke cannot be predicted with confidence. This is particularly true when the patient is seen early in the course of cerebral thrombosis. Often the course of cerebral thrombosis is progressive so the doctor is justified in being cautious with a patient who first appears to have suffered only a mild stroke. Progression of the stroke is most often due to increasing stenosis of the occluded artery by the thrombus. In some cases, the thrombus may extend along the vessel to block other arterial branches or prevent anastomotic flow from other vessels.

The degree of swelling (edema) that develops and its location can markedly influence the short-term prognosis (Figure 4-4). With large or small infarcts that are in certain specific locations, the edema causes such a rise in intracranial pressure that the displacement, or herniation, of brain tissue causes death after several days. In other cases, the edema may cause a worsening of symptoms for a period of two to four days. The survival of a patient who is comatose or stuperous from the outset is determined in large part by controlling the brain edema. Brain edema reaches its maximum in three or four days, then slowly subsides.

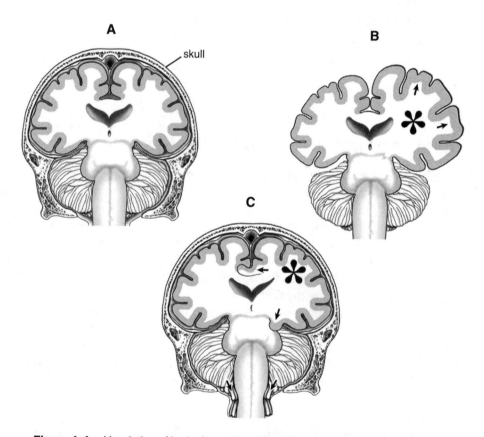

Figure 4-4.   Herniation of brain tissue is a potential consequence of brain edema. A, coronal section showing the normal adult brain within the confines of the non-expansible bony skull. B, edematous brain removed from the skull. If not confined by the skull, edema resulting from a stroke involving one hemisphere (indicated by asterisk) would cause that hemisphere to expand considerably. C, the skull prevents this expansion and forces soft brain tissue to herniate through normally available open passageways (arrows).

If the patient survives the completed stroke, the long-term prognosis usually favors improvement. The extent of the infarct is important. Recovery may begin in a day or two in patients with small infarcts and be virtually complete in a week or two. In patients with severe deficits, no meaningful improvement may occur even after months of intense rehabilitation. The longer the delay in the beginning of recovery, the poorer the prognosis becomes. Certain symptoms, such as language, speech, and walking, may continue to improve for years. It is believed by many that, in general, whatever deficits remain after 5 or 6 months will be permanent although their severity may decline over time. This opinion is not shared by all. Some studies have shown improvement to continue over extended periods, as long as 10 years.

As will become evident in the following section on stroke syndromes, strokes may result in an unbelievably wide array of clinical deficits ranging from complicated changes in personality to an inability to perceive sensations correctly or to move parts of the body. But there are some rather characteristic changes that occur in many strokes. One of these is a change in muscle tone. Muscle tone is the resistance muscle displays to passive stretch (lengthening) of a muscle, as when the doctor extends a patient's arm from an initially flexed position. Muscle tone is usually lost for a period of days or weeks following a stroke. Such loss is called a flaccid paralysis of muscle. The term *paralysis* refers to a loss of the ability to move a muscle voluntarily, that is, when the patient is asked to do so by a doctor or when the patient attempts to move an arm, leg, or toe on his own. The term *flaccid* refers to the loss of muscle tone.

After this initial flaccidity, muscle tone may gradually increase and eventually the increase may become marked. When the increase in muscle tone is marked, the paralysis then is called a spastic paralysis of muscle. The term *spastic* refers to the increase in muscle tone. In a spastic hemiplegia, the paralysis involves one-half of the body; the spasticity causes the arm to assume a flexed posture and the leg an extended posture. The early appearance of spasticity sometimes means a favorable prognosis.

In some patients, however, the hemiplegia remains flaccid and the arm dangles uselessly at the patient's side and the leg must be braced in order to support the patient's weight in standing. Bowel and bladder control may be lost initially, but usually return.

STROKE SYNDROMES

Each of the major cerebral arteries nourishes specific parts of the brain that have known functions. Because of this arterial branch-to-structure-to-function relation, involvement of particular arteries gives rise to signs and symptoms in different patients that are broadly similar. Thus, typical syndromes characterize cerebrovascular disease associated with a particular artery. However, the entire set of defects in a particular patient does *not* depend simply on the location of a lesion.

It is anatomically impossible to illustrate the entire pattern of vascularization of the brain in a single illustration and simultaneouly retain a clarity that facilitates understanding. Therefore, we have removed a section from a whole brain that contains a relatively small number of structures that have known functions. This is shown in Figure 4-5. The identified structures are nourished by the three major cere-

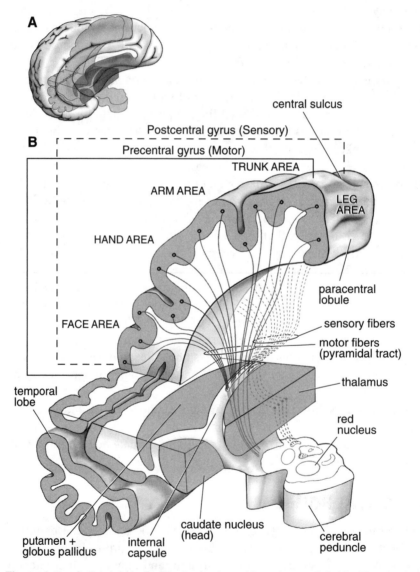

Figure 4-5.   A, the right half of the brain viewed from the medial side. The shaded area illustrates the section removed from the brain as shown in B and other figures. The size of the midbrain has been exaggerated. B, illustrates the relative positions of a number of important structures that may be damaged when particular blood vessels are involved in a stroke.

bral arteries derived from the internal carotid and vertebrobasilar systems. Various combinations of these structures can be damaged in a stroke to produce distinct syndromes. Figure 4-6 adds portions of the parietal, temporal, and occipital lobes to the section of Figure 4-5 along with the three cerebral arteries supplying these structures. The three arteries are the anterior cerebral artery (ACA), the middle cerebral

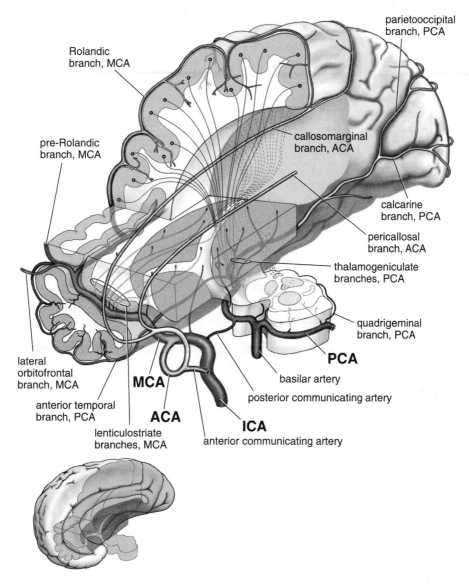

Figure 4-6. Sectioned brain (right half) illustrating known arteries supplying blood to the structures identified in Figure 4-5. Additional portions of the parietal and temporal lobes have been added as has the occipital lobe. Abbreviations: ACA, anterior cerebral artery; ICA, internal carotid artery; MCA, middle cerebral artery; PCA, posterior cerebral artery.

artery (MCA), and the posterior cerebral artery (PCA). Specific branches of each of these arteries are identified. Many subsequent figures, for example Figure 4-8, will then isolate particular portions of Figures 4-5 and 4-6 to illustrate a specific stroke syndrome.

The descriptions of the various syndromes that follow apply specifically to is-chemia and infarction, which occurs as a result of thrombosis and embolism. He-morrhagic strokes produce many of the same deficits but they usually involve the territory of more than just the damaged artery. This is due to the fact that the es-caped blood from a ruptured vessel does not respect the tissue boundaries nour-ished by an intact artery. Thus, a hemorrhage resulting from rupture of a surface artery may extend deeply into the substance of the brain. Further, because a hem-orrhage is a space-occupying lesion, it may exert pressure effects that compress vessels at some distance from the blood mass. Lastly, it is important to note that each syndrome is presented from the perspective of deficits that could appear with involvement of that artery. For obvious reasons, it is impossible to consider the wide variety of individual patient factors that might influence the nature and sever-ity of signs and symptoms.

Two types of arterial branches arise from the circle of Willis and the three ma-jor cerebral arteries. The first type is called a penetrating branch, and there are many. Penetrating branches (also called central or ganglionic) arise from the circle of Willis and from the proximal parts of the three cerebral arteries. There are many penetrating branches, for example, the lenticulostriate arteries and the thalamo-geniculate arteries (Figure 4-6). They dip perpendicularly into the substance of the brain and supply structures located deeply in the brain interior such as the dien-cephalon, basal ganglia (caudate nucleus, putamen, globus pallidus), and internal capsule (Figures 4-5, 4-6). The second type of arterial branch is called a cortical branch. Again, there are many, for example, the Rolandic artery and calcarine ar-tery (Figure 4-6). Cortical branches are larger than penetrating branches. Cortical branches divide repeatedly, finally giving off terminal branches of variable length that enter the brain. The shorter terminal branches supply the cerebral cortex, which forms the brain surface and has a thickness that varies from 1.5 to 4.5 mm depending upon location. The longer branches supply the immediately adjacent subcortical white matter. The territory of any artery, penetrating or cortical, may be involved in a stroke.

Each of the major cortical arteries is responsible for nourishing a specific region of the cerebral cortex. The region of cerebral cortex supplied by each artery is bro-ken down into a central territory and a peripheral territory (Figure 4-7). The central territory is the region of cortex for which the particular artery is the sole source of supply. No other artery contributes to the nourishment of nerve cells lying in the cen-tral territory of a major cortical artery. As a result, the central territory invariably un-dergoes extensive infarction when the vessel is severely occluded. In contrast, the peripheral territory of any of the major cerebral arteries also receives a blood supply

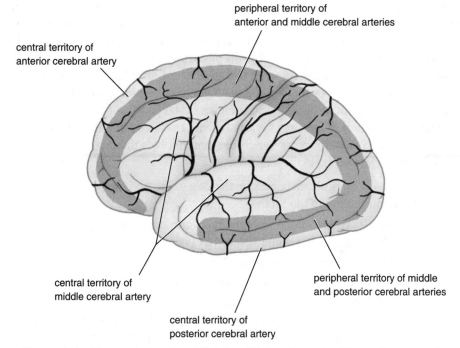

Figure 4-7. The central and peripheral territories of supply of the major cerebral arteries. See text for definitions. The left cerebral hemisphere is shown.

from another major artery. That is, the peripheral territory of an artery is the region of cortex that is also in the peripheral territory of one or more of the other major cerebral arteries. When a vessel is severely occluded, the peripheral territory usually is not as severely infarcted because it also receives a blood supply from another unoccluded vessel. Because the infarction in the peripheral territory is less extensive and fewer brain cells die, the resulting neurologic deficits would be correspondingly less severe.

The reason this distinction between central and peripheral territories is so important is that the central and peripheral territories of certain arteries supply areas of the cortex that receive information from, or control the movements of, distinct and different parts of the body. By noting the distribution and severity of neurologic deficits in different body parts, a neurologist can often determine the specific vessel that has been occluded.

The Middle Cerebral Artery

Syndrome of the Lenticulostriate Penetrating Branches. From its origin at the base of the brain, the middle cerebral artery (MCA) travels in a lateral direction toward the surface of the brain. As it does so, this main stem of the MCA gives off a number of penetrating branches. The penetrating branches are called the lenticulostriate arteries. The lenticulostriate arteries ascend perpendicularly to supply a number of structures including the clinically important internal capsule (posterior limb) (Figure 4-6). Atherothrombotic occlusion of certain of the lenticulostriate arteries illustrates the important principle that the location of an infarct is sometimes more important than its size. Lesions less than a cubic centimeter in size that involve the posterior limb of the internal capsule can cause a total paralysis of one-half the body.

The classic clinical syndrome associated with occlusion of the lenticulostriate arteries on one side is a pure motor syndrome that involves the face, arm, and leg in a spastic (capsular) hemiplegia (Figure 4-8).

- The spastic hemiplegia occurs on the side of the body opposite the lesion (the side contralateral to the infarct).
- The severity of involvement of the face, arm, and leg is equal and this is important in determining which artery has been occluded.
  - This equal impairment of the face, arm, and leg stands in contrast to the syndromes resulting from strokes involving cortical branches of the cerebral arteries.
    - Involvement of the cortical branches in a stroke results in the face, arm, and leg being affected to *different* degrees because of the distinction made previously between the central and peripheral territories of the cortical branches.
- There is a loss of voluntary control of the muscles of facial expression for the lower part of the face on the side contralateral to the lesion.
  - The patient will be unable to retract the corner of the mouth in a smile on one side when asked to do so, but would be able to wrinkle the forehead in a frown on that same side when asked to do so.
  - Although the patient cannot smile voluntarily (when asked) she may be able to contract those same muscles when she spontaneously laughs. (This is called emotional smiling.)
- Usually the spastic hemiplegia is relatively rapid in onset, but sometimes it evolves slowly over a period of two or three days.
- If the infarct is small, recovery may begin in hours, days, or weeks and progress to the point that within months there is little if any residual motor disability.
- Large infarcts in the territory of the lenticulostriate arteries may cause an enduring and severe spastic hemiplegia.

Additional penetrating branches in the same or opposite hemisphere may also become occluded. When these infarcts are small and the dead brain cells have been removed in the process of healing, a small cavity, called a lacune, is created (Figure 4-9). The clinical syndrome resulting from multiple small cavities is called the lacunar

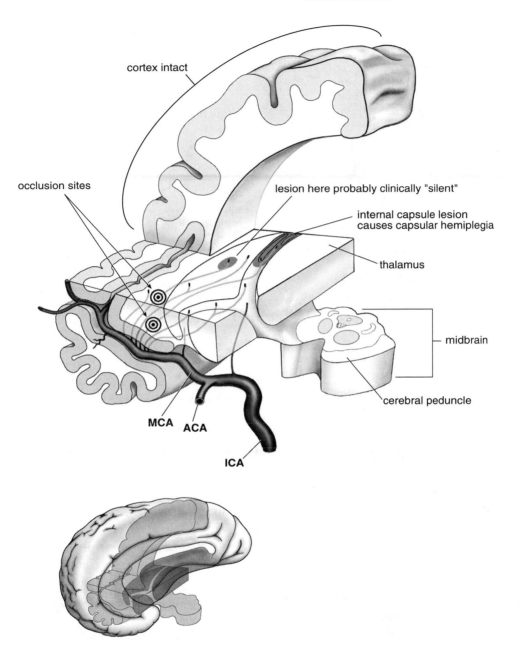

cortex intact

occlusion sites

lesion here probably clinically "silent"

internal capsule lesion
causes capsular hemiplegia

thalamus

midbrain

cerebral peduncle

MCA   ACA

ICA

Figure 4-8.   Occlusion of the lenticulostriate branches of the middle cerebral artery.
Blockage of these penetrating branches results in the pure motor syndrome of capsular (spastic) hemiplegia. The right half of the brain is shown. Abbreviations: ACA,
anterior cerebral artery; ICA, internal carotid artery; MCA, middle cerebral artery.

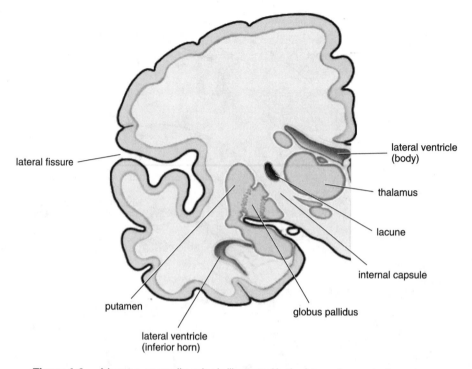

Figure 4-9.   A lacune, or small cavity, is illustrated in the internal capsule. Lacunes are produced when dead brain cells are removed after a small artery has become occluded.

state. There is no single, uniform syndrome characterizing the lacunar state because the neurologic deficits can vary widely depending on the specific locations of the lacunes. Besides the internal capsule, the lenticulostriate arteries nourish additional brain structures including the putamen, most of the caudate nucleus, and parts of the globus pallidus. Lacunes may be located in any or all of these structures.

One known syndrome produced by *multiple* lacunar infarcts is pseudobulbar palsy. The usual history of a patient who develops pseudobulbar palsy is that he suffered lacunar infarcts involving the internal capsule on one side of the brain at an earlier point in time. The part of the internal capsule involved in pseudobulbar palsy carries a set of nerve fibers called corticobulbar fibers. Corticobulbar fibers connect the cerebral cortex with nerve cells in the brain stem that control the oral and facial muscles. It is important to note that the oral, facial, laryngeal and pharyngeal muscles are controlled by corticobulbar fibers from *both* sides of the brain. As a result, infarcts involving corticobulbar fibers on just one side will not produce a permanent impairment in speech or swallowing (Figure 4-10). The presence of continuing atherosclerosis and hypertension, however, lead to the later development of lacunar infarcts affecting corticobulbar fibers in the opposite internal capsule. The patient now has sustained dam-

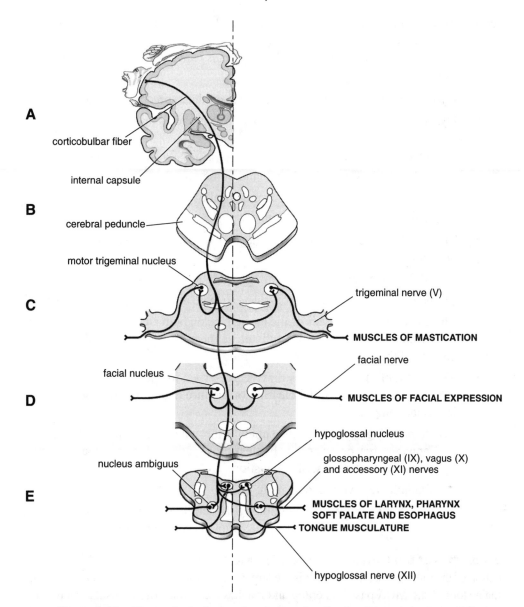

A

corticobulbar fiber

internal capsule

B

cerebral peduncle

motor trigeminal nucleus

C

trigeminal nerve (V)

MUSCLES OF MASTICATION

facial nerve

facial nucleus

D

MUSCLES OF FACIAL EXPRESSION

hypoglossal nucleus

glossopharyngeal (IX), vagus (X) and accessory (XI) nerves

nucleus ambiguus

E

MUSCLES OF LARYNX, PHARYNX SOFT PALATE AND ESOPHAGUS
TONGUE MUSCULATURE

hypoglossal nerve (XII)

Figure 4-10.   The corticobulbar system innervating the cranial nerve motor nuclei that control the oral and facial muscles. A, frontal section through the precentral gyrus of the cerebral cortex of the right cerebral hemisphere. B, transverse section through the midbrain. C, transverse section through the midpons. D, transverse section through the lower pons. E, transverse section through the midmedulla. Beginning in C, note that the fibers of the corticobulbar system arising from just one side of the cerebral cortex supply cranial nerve motor nuclei on both sides of the brain stem (the nuclei are bilaterally innervated).

age to the corticobulbar fibers in both the right and left internal capsules and this bilateral damage produces the syndrome of pseudobulbar palsy.

The symptoms characterizing pseudobulbar palsy are numerous. The full array of symptoms include:

- Dysarthria in which the patient is unable to produce speech (articulate) normally.
- Dysphonia in which the patient is unable to properly make voiced sounds by vibration of the vocal cords.
  - □ If the patient is asked to produce (phonate) a prolonged vowel, such as "ah," there is more air than sound in the vowel.
- Dysphagia in which the patient cannot swallow properly.
- The patient cannot move his tongue.
- There is a spastic paralysis of the muscles of mastication so the patient cannot chew.
  - □ This is accompanied by an exaggerated jaw jerk reflex.
- The patient cannot elevate the soft palate so there is a nasal regurgitation of food.
- There is a spastic paralysis of the entire face on both sides so the patient cannot wrinkle the forehead, forcefully close the eyes, or elevate and retract the corners of the mouth in a voluntary smile.
- Movement of all the muscles may be preserved in spontaneous movements such as yawning, coughing, clearing of the throat, and in spasmodic (pathologic) laughing and crying.
  - □ In pathologic laughing, the patient is thrown into gales of laughter for no apparent reason or at the slightest provocation. Hilarious laughter may continue to the point of exhaustion.
  - □ Pathologic crying occurs more often.
    - ♦ For example, just mentioning the family in conversation may cause the patient to go into a bout of uncontrollable crying.

Syndromes of the Cortical Branches. The MCA is considered to be the direct continuation of the internal carotid artery. It is the largest of the three major cerebral arteries. The main stem of the MCA passes laterally and reaches the surface of the insula where it divides into a number of branches. Collectively, these branches form what is called the Sylvian triangle (Figure 4-11). The Sylvian triangle is an important landmark when blood vessels of the brain are visualized during cerebral angiography. The cortical branches of the MCA supply most of the lateral surface of each of the brain's two cerebral hemispheres.

Although structurally similar, the brain's right and left cerebral hemispheres are not equivalent functionally. One hemisphere is designated as the dominant hemisphere, the other the nondominant hemisphere. Originally, this distinction was based on the fact that most of our language abilities are controlled by just one hemisphere, which was called the dominant hemisphere. In most people (over 90 percent), the

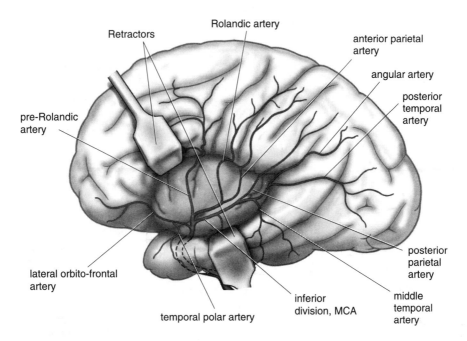

Figure 4-11. Insular arteries. Portions of the frontal and parietal lobes have been retracted to show how branches of the middle cerebral artery are distributed over the surface of the insula to form the sylvian triangle. After dividing, the branches reach the lateral surface of the hemisphere via the lateral (sylvian) fissure. The left cerebral hemisphere is shown. Abbreviation: MCA, middle cerebral artery.

dominant hemisphere is the left. Since this original distinction, other abilities have been shown to be controlled primarily by one or the other of the two hemispheres, but the dominant-nondominant distinction based on language still remains. The importance of this distinction is that strokes occurring in equivalent areas in the left and right hemispheres may result in qualitatively different neurological deficits.

In addition to the dominance distinction, different parts of a single cerebral hemisphere are distinguished by different numbers. Early in the twentieth century, the cerebral cortex of each hemisphere was divided into 52 different areas by the neuroanatomist Korbinian Brodmann. The basis for distinguishing one cortical area from another is of no immediate concern to us. What is important is the fact that different areas have come to be associated with different functions. Brodmann's mapping system is still in widespread use so neurologists will refer to a stroke having affected, for example, Brodmann's areas (BAs) 44 and 45 in the dominant or nondominant hemisphere.

The main stem of the MCA on the surface of the insula divides into two main cortical divisions: a superior division and an inferior division. Each division, in turn, is composed of a number of branches that individually supply different areas of the cortex with specific Brodmann's numbers. Figure 4-12 shows the branches of the MCA. Figure 4-13 illustrates the functional areas of the cerebral cortex and their Brodmann's numbers supplied by the various branches of the MCA.

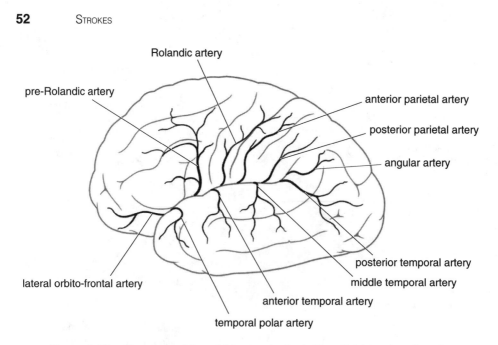

Rolandic artery

pre-Rolandic artery

anterior parietal artery

posterior parietal artery

angular artery

posterior temporal artery

middle temporal artery

lateral orbito-frontal artery

anterior temporal artery

temporal polar artery

Figure 4-12. Branches of the middle cerebral artery on the lateral surface (convexity) of the left hemisphere. These branches arise from either the superior or inferior division of the artery.

There are three clinically important branches of the superior division. A pre-Rolandic branch supplies the premotor cortex, a region of the cortex responsible for turning the head and deviating the eyes laterally to the contralateral side (BA 8), and, in the dominant hemisphere only, the motor speech-language area of Broca (also called the anterior speech area, BAs 44 and 45). A Rolandic branch supplies the primary motor area (BA 4) of the precentral gyrus and some of the primary sensory area of the postcentral gyrus. An anterior parietal (post-Rolandic) branch supplies most of the primary sensory cortex of the postcentral gyrus (BAs 3, 2, 1).

Branches of the inferior division of the MCA are named after the cortical area supplied. These include: anterior, middle, and posterior temporal branches; a posterior parietal branch; and an angular branch. In the dominant hemisphere (usually the left), a number of these branches contribute to the supply of the sensory speech-language area of Wernicke (BAs 22, 40, 39) (also called the posterior speech area). In the nondominant hemisphere (usually the right), these same branches contribute to the supply of an area of cortex that is responsible for visuospatial functions. Such visuospatial functions include the ability to understand and use visual representations and spatial relationships in learning and in performing a task such as dressing or drawing a three-dimensional object.

Main Stem Syndrome. Occlusion of the main stem of the MCA before it gives off any branches blocks the flow of blood into the penetrating lenticulostriate arteries as well as into the superficial cortical branches belonging to both the superior and infe-

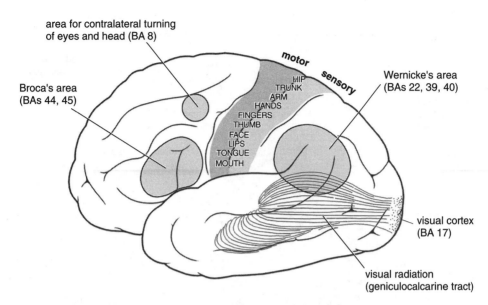

Figure 4-13. Location of areas in the left cerebral hemisphere that when damaged produce focal neurological deficits. In the majority of people, the speech-language areas of Broca and Wernicke are located only in the left (dominant) hemisphere. Corresponding areas in the nondominant (usually right) hemisphere have different functions. The Brodmann's numbers associated with the cortical areas (BAs) are indicated. Parts of the body represented in the precentral (motor) and postcentral (sensory) gyri are indicated. Abbreviation: BA, Brodmann's area.

rior divisions (Figure 4-14). The resultant syndrome would be a summation of the lenticulostriate and cortical branch syndromes. Figure 4-15 shows the large cortical area affected by occlusion of the main stem of the MCA.

- The equal involvement of the face, arm, and leg on the contralateral side in a spastic hemiplegia is produced by occlusion of the lenticulostriate arteries and a resultant infarction in the posterior limb of the internal capsule.

- The head and eyes deviate toward the side of the lesion due to destruction of BA 8.

- The sensory impairment over the contralateral *face* and *arm* (hemianesthesia) is due to infarction of BAs 3, 1, 2 of the postcentral gyrus. On standard tests of sensation, the patient would exhibit:

  □ Impairment or loss of the ability to distinguish objects by their size, shape, and texture (astereognosis).

  □ Impairment or loss of ability to identify letters, numbers, or shapes drawn on the skin surface (agraphesthesia).

  □ Impairment or loss of the sense of position and movement.

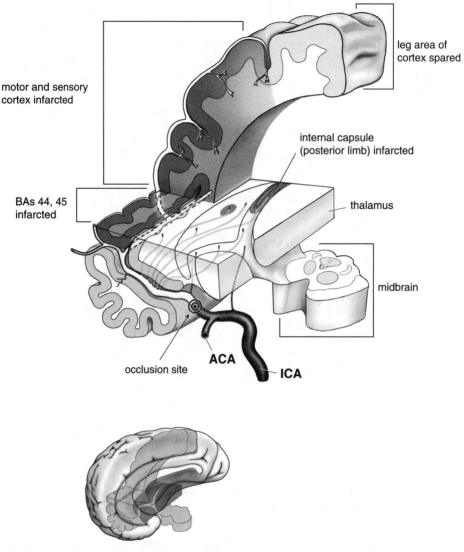

motor and sensory
cortex infarcted

leg area of
cortex spared

internal capsule
(posterior limb) infarcted

thalamus

BAs 44, 45
infarcted

midbrain

occlusion site

ACA

ICA

Figure 4-14. Occlusion of the main stem of the middle cerebral artery results in infarction of brain tissue supplied by both the penetrating and cortical branches of the artery (shaded areas of the brain). Cortical areas in addition to those illustrated also will be infarcted. The right half of the brain is shown. Abbreviations: ACA, anterior cerebral artery; BA, Brodmann's area; ICA, internal carotid artery.

- □ Impairment or loss of the ability to discriminate two points simultaneously applied to the skin surface (two-point discrimination).

- □ Impairment or loss of the ability to localize the point on the body stimulated by touch (point localization).

- □ Variable changes in touch, pain, and temperature sense.

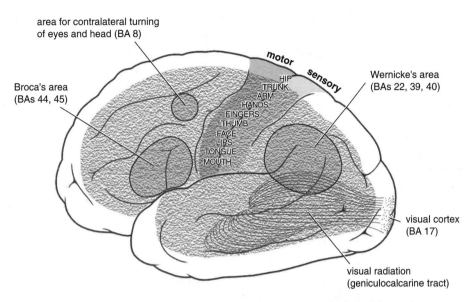

area for contralateral turning
of eyes and head (BA 8)

Broca's area
(BAs 44, 45)

motor

sensory

HIP
TRUNK
ARM
HANDS
FINGERS
THUMB
FACE
LIPS
TONGUE
MOUTH

Wernicke's area
(BAs 22, 39, 40)

visual cortex
(BA 17)

visual radiation
(geniculocalcarine tract)

Figure 4-15. Area of the left hemisphere infarcted by occlusion of the main stem of the left middle cerebral artery (textured area). The infarcted area includes specific cortical regions (dark shading) whose damage results in the prominent signs and symptoms associated with such a stroke. Abbreviation: BA, Brodmann's area.

- The patient will be blind to visual stimuli in the contralateral half of the same visual field in each eye (homonymous hemianopsia) due to infarction of the white matter of the optic radiation in the temporal lobe.

- If the main stem of the dominant hemisphere is occluded there will, in addition to the previous, be a global (mixed) aphasia.
  - □ The patient can say only a few words (hypofluent).
  - □ The global aphasic may understand a few words or phrases, but there is a gross defect in comprehension such that the patient cannot carry out a series of simple commands.
  - □ The patient cannot read, write, or repeat what is said to him.
  - □ These language deficits may not improve at all or may improve very little over a period of months or years.
    - ♦ Usually, the patient never regains effective communication.

- When the main stem of the nondominant hemisphere is involved, rather than the global aphasia, the patient will exhibit contralateral visuospatial neglect in which visual stimuli on the left side are neglected. See inferior division occlusions, on p. 59, for the symptoms of visuospatial neglect.

Cortical branches of the MCA are most often occluded by emboli originating in the heart (cardiogenic). It should be noted that the cortical branches of the *left* MCA are a more frequent site for the lodgment of emboli than are branches of the right MCA. This is because the left common carotid artery is a direct off-shoot from the arch of the aorta. An embolus entering the MCA may lodge in the superior division, the inferior division, or in their individual branches.

Superior Division Syndrome. Superior division occlusions result in the following symptoms:

- Sensory and motor deficits in the contralateral face and arm due to infarction of the pre- and postcentral gyri (Figure 4-16).
- The degree to which the hand is involved in the sensory and motor deficits depends on the extent of collateral circulation the hand representation in the cortex receives from the unoccluded anterior cerebral artery.
  - Thus, only the central territory of the superior division might be involved, in which case the hand would show no deficits.
  - If the entire territory (central and peripheral) were involved, the hand would display sensory and motor deficits.
- The sensory deficits take the form of
  - Astereognosis
  - Loss of or impaired graphesthesia (agraphesthesia)
  - Impaired sense of position and movement
  - Failure of point (tactile) localization and two-point discrimination
  - Variable changes in touch, pain, and temperature sensation
- Infarction in the dominant hemisphere causes at first a global aphasia that soon changes to a motor (expressive, or Broca's) aphasia.

A motor aphasia is due to infarction in frontal lobe BAs 44 and 45 (Figure 4-17). A motor aphasia is characterized by:

- The use of a lower than normal number of words (hypofluent).
- The use of informative, key words (action verbs and nouns) with simplified grammar.
- An inability to retrieve from memory words the patient wants to use (a word-finding problem) resulting in hesitant speech with pauses.
- Difficulty with the initiation and production of speech. Some patients have to expend considerable effort just to start talking.
- Loss of the normal melody, rhythm, and inflection patterns in speech (loss of prosody, or aprosody).
- Normal comprehension of written and spoken words.

An embolic occlusion that is limited to one of the branches of the superior division would result in a more restricted set of the previous symptoms.

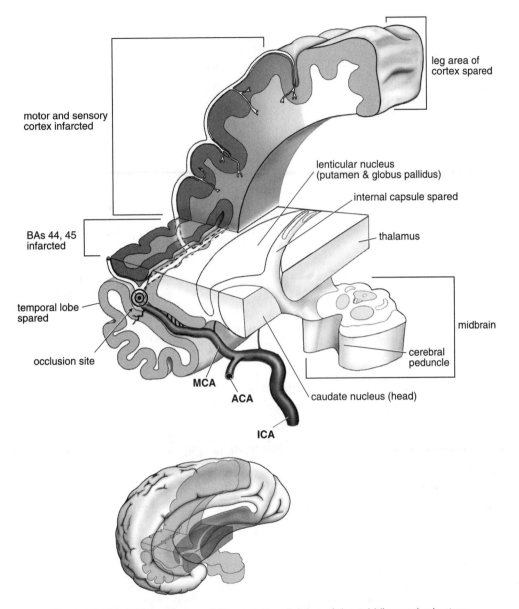

leg area of
cortex spared

motor and sensory
cortex infarcted

lenticular nucleus
(putamen & globus pallidus)

internal capsule spared

thalamus

BAs 44, 45
infarcted

temporal lobe
spared

midbrain

occlusion site

cerebral
peduncle

MCA

ACA

caudate nucleus (head)

ICA

Figure 4-16.   With occlusion of the superior division of the middle cerebral artery
(MCA) only the cerebral cortex and subjacent white matter are infarcted (shaded),
not the territory supplied by the penetrating branches of the artery. The inferior division of the MCA is not shown. The right half of the brain is illustrated. Abbreviations:
ACA, anterior cerebral artery; BAs, Brodmann's areas; ICA, internal carotid artery.

- Involvement of the pre-Rolandic branch in the dominant hemisphere may result in an isolated Broca's aphasia.
- Occlusion of the Rolandic branch may result in a spastic hemiplegia (paralysis) involving the contralateral face and arm and dysarthria, but no aphasia.

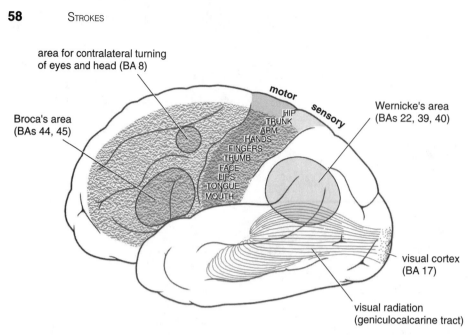

Figure 4-17. Area of the left hemisphere infarcted by occlusion of the left superior division of the middle cerebral artery (textured area). Note that the damage is confined to the frontal lobe and postcentral gyrus of the parietal lobe. Abbreviation: BA, Brodmann's area.

- Occlusion of the anterior parietal (post-Rolandic) branch would result in contralateral sensory deficits in the face and arm.

Inferior Division Syndrome. Inferior division occlusions occur less often than do occlusions of the superior division. Inferior division occlusions are also almost always due to cardiogenic embolism. Figure 4-18 shows the cortical areas affected by occlusion of the inferior division of the MCA. Symptoms of inferior division occlusion are different depending upon whether the left or right hemisphere is involved:

- Lesions involving the dominant left hemisphere typically result in a sensory (receptive, or Wernicke's) aphasia. A sensory aphasia is due to damage to BAs 40 and 39.
  - □ The patient uses an excessive number of words (hyperfluent).
    - ♦ Many relational words that do not carry significant meaning are used.
  - □ The patient may substitute incorrect syllables for correct ones and incorrect words for correct ones.
  - □ The patient may "invent" new words that have no meaning (neologism).
  - □ There is a word-finding problem, usually less severe than in Broca's aphasia.
  - □ Speech is produced effortlessly.
  - □ Prosody is normal.

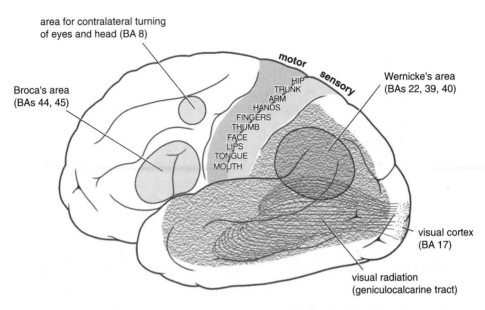

Figure 4-18. Area of the left hemisphere infarcted by occlusion of the inferior division of the middle cerebral artery (textured area). Note that the damage is confined to the posterior portion of the parietal lobe and the temporal lobe. Abbreviation: BA, Brodmann's area.

- □ Comprehension of spoken and written language is deficient.
- A contralateral homonymous hemianopsia occurs with lesions involving either the right or left hemisphere.
- When damage involves BAs 40 and 39 in the right, nondominant hemisphere, a contralateral visuospatial neglect occurs. The term visuospatial neglect covers a number of symptoms and signs. These deficits also have been called asomatoagnosia and amorphosynthesis.
  - □ The patient neglects the left side of the body in dressing and grooming. Some patients feel that the left side of their body has disappeared.
  - □ The patient may be unable to manipulate articles of clothing properly so that they are unable to put on a coat when one sleeve has been turned inside out (dressing apraxia).
  - □ The patient may shave only the right half of the face, apply lipstick only to the right side of the lips, or comb only the right side of the hair.
  - □ The patient may fail to draw the left half of the face of a clock, or fail to draw the petals on the left side of a flower.
  - □ In assembling a set of blocks to duplicate a design shown to the patient (such as a three-dimensional triangle), the patient may neglect the left half of the design and assemble only the right half (constructional apraxia).

- ☐ When right hemisphere lesions involving the motor area of the frontal lobe extend into the parietal lobe, the patient may be unaware of, or indifferent to, the paralyzed left arm.

  - ♦ In extreme form, a patient shown her paralyzed arm may deny that it is hers, state that it belongs to someone else, and even attempt to throw it aside. This deficit is called anosoagnosia.

The Anterior Cerebral Artery

Occlusion of the anterior cerebral artery (ACA) is much less common than occlusion of the larger middle cerebral and internal carotid arteries. One reason is that the ACA may simply be less susceptible to the development of atherosclerosis. This is suggested by the fact that at postmortem examination atherosclerotic plaques are found less frequently in the ACA than in other major vessels.

In addition, even when one ACA is occluded, the ACA territory potentially can receive collateral circulation from a number of sources: (1) from the large MCA of the same side via end-to-end meningeal anastomoses; (2) from the ACA of the opposite side via meningeal anastomoses over the surface of the corpus callosum; and (3) from the opposite ACA via the anterior communicating artery. In the latter case, occlusion of the stem of the ACA before (proximal to) its connection with the anterior communicating artery may not cause symptoms because the ACA distal to the occlusion receives sufficient blood from the *opposite* ACA over the anterior communicating artery (Figure 4-19).

The cortical branches of the ACA supply the anterior three-fourths of the medial surface of the cerebral hemisphere as well as the anterior four-fifths of the corpus callosum. The corpus callosum is the massive band of fibers that interconnects the two cerebral hemispheres allowing them to communicate with one another. Named cortical branches supply the medial and orbital surfaces of the frontal lobe, the frontal pole, the medial surface of the parietal lobe, and a strip of the lateral surface of the cerebral hemisphere along the superior border (Figure 4-20). Figure 4-21 shows important functional areas supplied by the ACA.

Syndrome of Unilateral Occlusion. Unilateral occlusion of one ACA distal to the anterior communicating artery produces motor and sensory symptoms that are most severe in the contralateral lower extremity with minor involvement of the contralateral upper extremity and no involvement of the face (Figure 4-22). The resulting syndrome potentially could include:

- Spastic paralysis that is more severe in the foot and leg than in the thigh.
- The degree of involvement of the arm is variable because the arm is represented in a cortical area that is located in the peripheral territory of the MCA as well as the ACA.

  - ☐ The degree of arm involvement depends on the adequacy of supply to the arm area received from end-to-end meningeal anastomoses with the MCA.

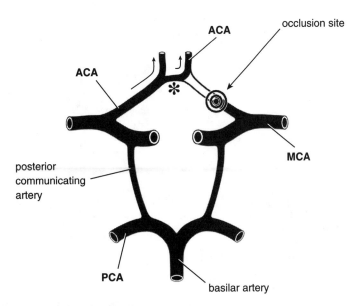

Figure 4-19.   Ventral view of the circle of Willis. When the left anterior cerebral artery is occluded as shown, the anterior cerebral artery distal to the occlusion may still receive adequate blood from the *right* anterior cerebral artery over the anterior communicating artery located above the asterisk. Abbreviations: ACA, anterior cerebral artery; MCA, middle cerebral artery; PCA, posterior cerebral artery.

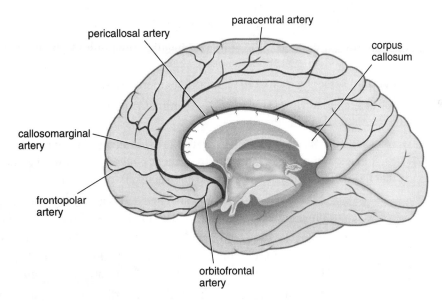

Figure 4-20.   The medial surface of the right cerebral hemisphere is shown. Cortical branches of the anterior cerebral artery supply the anterior three-fourths of the medial surface and the anterior portions of the corpus callosum.

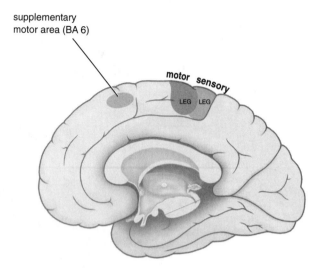

Figure 4-21. Medial view of the right hemisphere showing the location of several functional areas in the territory of the anterior cerebral artery. Abbreviation: BA, Brodmann's area.

- The sensory loss may be mild or even absent in some cases. When present, the sensory impairment or loss involves discriminative sensation:
  - Impairment or loss of the ability to identify letters, numbers, or shapes drawn on the skin surface (agraphesthesia).
  - Impairment or loss of the sense of position or movement.
  - Impairment or loss of the ability to discriminate two points simultaneously applied to the skin surface (two-point discrimination).
  - Impairment or loss of the ability to localize the point on the leg stimulated by touch (point localization).
  - Variable changes in touch, pain, and temperature sense.
- Infarctions in the territory of the ACA sometimes produce a syndrome known as the alien hand syndrome (AHS).
  - All patients with AHS exhibit actions of an extremity that are experienced as involuntary and often contrary to the patient's stated intention. The normal hand usually attempts to restrain the alien hand. Two forms of AHS exist.
    - Frontal AHS occurs in the dominant hand and is associated with reflexive grasping, impulsive groping, and compulsive manipulation of tools.
      - Frontal AHS results from infarction to the supplementary motor cortex, anterior cingulate gyrus, and medial prefrontal cortex of the dominant hemisphere and the anterior corpus callosum.
    - Callosal AHS is characterized mainly by conflict between the actions of the two hands and requires only infarction of the corpus callosum.
- Small lesions limited to the supplementary motor area (SMA) can cause a pure disorder of speech initiation (Figure 4-21).

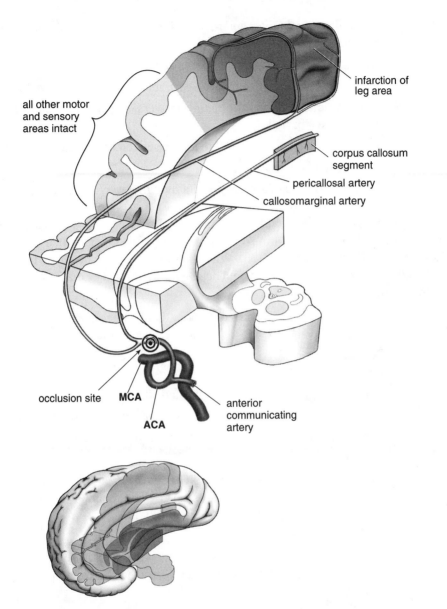

all other motor
and sensory
areas intact

infarction of
leg area

corpus callosum
segment

pericallosal artery

callosomarginal artery

occlusion site   **MCA**

ACA

anterior
communicating
artery

Figure 4-22. Occlusion of the right anterior cerebral artery at the site shown results in infarction of the cerebral cortex and subjacent white matter as well as the corpus callosum (shaded). The right half of the brain is shown. Abbreviations: ACA, anterior cerebral artery; MCA, middle cerebral artery.

- Transcortical motor aphasia or other unusual subcortical aphasias may result from larger lesions in the white matter deep to the SMA, above and lateral to the frontal horn of the lateral ventricle following occlusion of the penetrating branches of the ACA in the dominant (left) hemisphere.

- The transcortical motor aphasia develops *after* a period of muteness that may last for days to weeks.
- The patient has limited spontaneous speech.
- There may be a limited ability to name objects and to compose word lists.
- Major deficits occur in formulating answers to open-ended questions and in narrative storytelling.
- The patient retains the ability to repeat spoken and written sentences.
- Articulation is normal.
- Auditory comprehension is good, although it may be impaired initially.

Syndrome of Bilateral Occlusion. Maximal deficits are produced with bilateral infarctions when blood flow in both ACAs is arrested. This occurs when both ACAs arise from one ACA stem (Figure 4-23). When this stem becomes occluded infarctions of the medial frontal-parietal areas of both hemispheres occur. The resultant syndrome potentially can include:

- A change in personality and affect (mood) that is thought to be due to infarction of the medial and orbital surfaces of the frontal lobe.
  - The patient is euphoric and has a lack of concern for the present or the future.
  - The patient may exhibit a childlike and silly attitude.
  - Erotic behavior, lewd remarks, and sexual exhibitionism may occur.
  - The patient may make inappropriate jokes and caustic or facetious remarks.
  - Outbursts of irritability are common.
  - These outbursts of excitation and euphoria appear episodically and are superimposed on a background of apathy and reduction in spontaneous movement, spoken words and thought (abulia).
- Urinary incontinence may occur.
- There may be an apraxia of the nondominant (left), nonparalyzed hand (sympathetic apraxia) such that the patient cannot use the hand appropriately when asked to do so.
  - This is thought to be due to involvement of the fibers of the corpus callosum.
- Both lower extremities may exhibit cortical sensory and motor deficits.

The Internal Carotid Artery

The neurologic deficits resulting from atherothrombotic occlusion of the internal carotid artery are more variable than with occlusion of any other vessel. In some

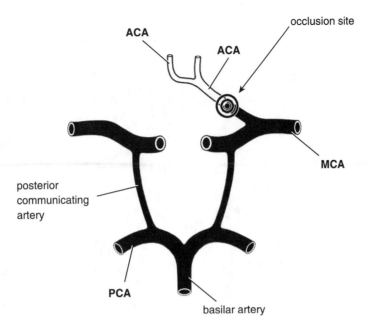

Figure 4-23. Ventral view of the circle of Willis. When both anterior cerebral arteries arise from one ACA stem, occlusion of that stem results in an infarction involving both sides of the brain (bilateral infarctions). Abbreviations: ACA, anterior cerebral artery; MCA, middle cerebral artery; PCA, posterior cerebral artery.

cases, occlusion of one internal carotid artery may not produce any deficits at all if the collateral supply from other vessels is adequate. In other cases, occlusion may result in a massive infarction of the anterior two-thirds of the entire cerebral hemisphere and lead to death in a few days. As noted earlier, favored locations for stenosis in this system are at the bifurcation of the common carotid artery into the external and internal carotid arteries and at the carotid siphon. The branches of the internal carotid artery in their order of occurrence are the ophthalmic artery, the posterior communicating artery, the anterior choroidal artery, the ACA, and the MCA (Figure 4-24).

The presence of occlusions in the common and internal carotid arteries can be evaluated directly in contrast to other cerebral arteries where occlusion is determined either by the resulting clinical deficits or by diagnostic imaging procedures such as MRI or CT scanning. Direct evaluation is done by placing a stethoscope on certain sites in the neck and listening for sounds generated as a result of the turbulent flow of blood in the arteries. Turbulence is caused by a narrowing (stenosis) of the vessel lumen. The sound is called a bruit (French—noise). When bruit is heard at the angle of the jaw, the area of stenosis and turbulent flow is at the bifurcation of the common and internal carotid arteries (that is, in the carotid sinus) (Figure 4-25). When bruit

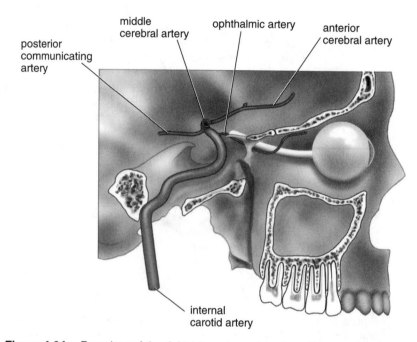

posterior
communicating
artery

middle
cerebral artery

ophthalmic artery

anterior
cerebral artery

internal
carotid artery

Figure 4-24. Branches of the right internal carotid artery. The anterior choroidal artery is not shown

is heard lower in the neck, just above the clavicle, the stenosis is in the common carotid or subclavian arteries. Stenoses that are not tight enough or those that are too tight may generate no bruit at all so the absence of bruit is of little significance.

Monocular Blindness. The ophthalmic artery nourishes the optic nerve and retina of the eye. In about 25 percent of the cases that develop symptomatic carotid occlusion, the stroke is preceded by episodes of transient monocular blindness due to occlusion of the ophthalmic artery. The episodes of monocular blindness are referred to as amaurosis fugax. Many of these episodes develop quickly (10 seconds or so). Symptoms may include:

- A unilateral graying out of vision of the eye, often spreading from the periphery to the center of the field of vision.
- This is followed by either total blindness or a sense of seeing only shadows through a thick gray mist.
- The episodes generally last for seconds, rarely for more than a few minutes.
- The episode clears slowly and smoothly.

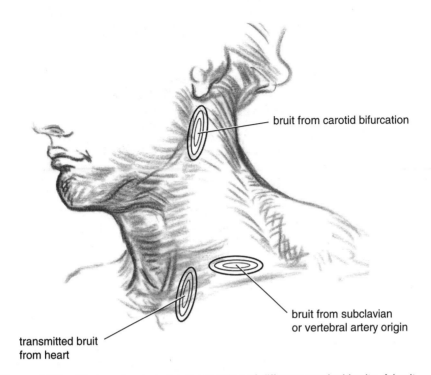

bruit from carotid bifurcation

bruit from subclavian
or vertebral artery origin

transmitted bruit
from heart

Figure 4-25. Diagram to show the localization of different cervical bruits. A bruit high up under the angle of the jaw results from stenosis at the carotid bifurcation. Bruits above the clavicle are caused by occlusions at the origin of either the subclavian or vertebral arteries.

Carotid Border Syndrome. One of the more common patterns of carotid artery insufficiency occurs with occlusion of one carotid artery and is called the carotid border syndrome. The internal carotid artery must be occluded by at least 70 percent in order to produce the carotid border syndrome. With this degree of occlusion, blood flow in the artery distal to the occlusion is decreased significantly but is not eliminated. In this situation, the peripheral territories of both the middle and anterior cerebral arteries represent the zone of maximal ischemia. This zone called the watershed area (Figure 4-26).

Maximal ischemia occurs in the watershed area because it requires the greatest pressure for blood to reach the terminal ends of the two arteries where the vessels have the smallest diameter. The area of maximal ischemia is also referred to as the border zone between the middle and anterior cerebral arteries, hence the clinical name of carotid border syndrome. The portion of the body represented in the pre- and postcentral gyri belonging to this border zone is the hand. The border zone is also the most

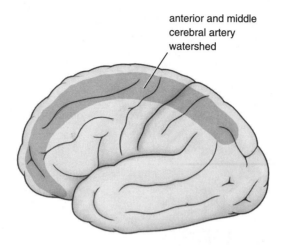

anterior and middle
cerebral artery
watershed

A

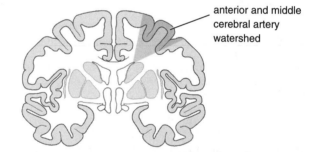

anterior and middle
cerebral artery
watershed

B

Figure 4-26. A, the watershed area on the lateral surface of the left hemisphere formed by the middle and anterior cerebral arteries (shaded). The watershed area is in the peripheral territories of each artery and represents the zone of maximal ischemia with stenosis of the internal carotid artery on that side. The peripheral territory of the posterior cerebral artery is not shown. B, coronal section of the brain showing the watershed area of the anterior and middle cerebral arteries (shaded). Note that in addition to the cortex, the subjacent white matter also is infarcted.

vulnerable cortical area in cases of transient ischemia attacks with stenosis of the internal carotid artery.

The symptoms in the carotid border syndrome include numbness and weakness of the contralateral hand.

MCA Syndrome. As a general rule, occlusion of the internal carotid artery most often produces ischemia of the cerebral cortex within the peripheral and central territories of supply of the MCA. Infarction of the cortex in the area supplied by the ACA is less likely to occur because the ACA is more likely to receive adequate collateral supply from other vessels. With increasing stenosis of the internal carotid artery, the zone of ischemia extends from the border zone into the area of central supply of the MCA. In this situation, additional symptoms occur (Figure 4-15):

- In addition to the hand and arm, the face becomes involved.
- The face will be numb and there will be a spastic paralysis of the muscles of the lower half of the face.
    - □ The facial deficits are on the side opposite the lesion.
- When the dominant hemisphere is involved in the infarct, an aphasia results.
    - □ The aphasia is most often an expressive (motor, Broca's) aphasia.
    - □ There may, however, be a sensory (receptive, Wernicke's) aphasia or a mixed aphasia if both the anterior and posterior speech areas are involved.
- When the nondominant hemisphere is involved, rather than an aphasia, there will be unilateral visuospatial neglect.

The Posterior Cerebral Artery

The posterior cerebral arteries (PCAs) are a part of the vertebral-basilar system, the second of the two major systems that supply blood to the brain. In about 70 percent of autopsied brains the PCAs originate as the direct continuations of the basilar artery upon its bifurcation (Figure 4-27). As a result, occlusive disease of the basilar (or vertebral) artery may result in the development of symptoms in the territories of both PCAs.

Occlusion of the PCA can produce a greater variety of clinical effects than can occlusion of any other artery. This is because of the complexity of organization of the brain regions it supplies: the upper brain stem and parts of the temporal and occipital lobes. The upper brain stem is crowded with important structures that produce easily recognized symptoms. The inferior and medial parts of the temporal and occipital lobe also contain cortical areas that produce a variety of clearly observable symptoms when infarcted.

The extent of the infarction from PCA occlusion will be determined by several factors. The first is the specific organization of the circle of Willis. The second is the extent of collateral flow into the territory of the PCA through border zone meningeal anastomoses with the ACA and MCA.

Syndromes of the Penetrating Branches. The penetrating branches of the PCA supply the rostral portion of the midbrain and thalamus (Figure 4-28). A number of syndromes follow occlusion of these penetrating branches. The symptoms characterizing these syndromes may occur in various combinations and also be associated with other neurologic signs.

Thalamic Syndrome (of Dejerine and Roussy). This syndrome results from occlusion of the thalamocingulate branches that supply the posterior half of the thalamus (Figure 4-29). The syndrome consists of three components that occur in variable proportion in different patients: hemianesthesia, sensory ataxia, and thalamic pain.

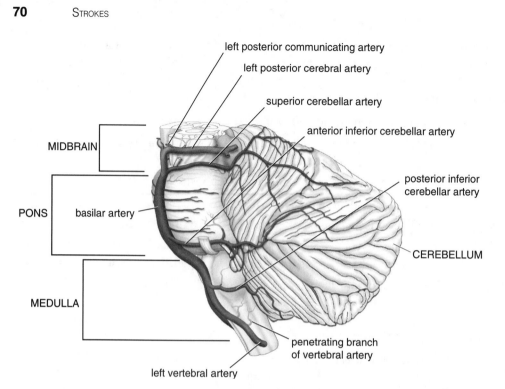

left posterior communicating artery

left posterior cerebral artery

superior cerebellar artery

anterior inferior cerebellar artery

posterior inferior cerebellar artery

CEREBELLUM

MIDBRAIN

PONS

basilar artery

MEDULLA

penetrating branch of vertebral artery

left vertebral artery

Figure 4-27. The posterior cerebral arteries arise from the bifurcation of the basilar artery. They are a part of the vertebral-basilar system.

- Hemianesthesia is a severe, and sometimes total, loss of somatic sensation on the opposite side of the head and body.

- After a variable period of time sensation begins to return and the patient then develops thalamic pain and an exaggerated subjective response to pain that may continue after the stimulus has stopped (hyperpathia).

  □ The pain may be triggered by stimuli that normally are not painful, such as touch, or may even occur spontaneously.

- Paresthesias also develop.

  □ Paresthesias (dysesthesias) are unnatural sensations and may occur spontaneously or in response to stimulation.

- Sensory ataxia expresses itself as uncoordinated movements.

  □ It is due to the fact that the brain is deprived of proprioceptive information about the position and movement of the parts of the body it is trying to control.

Amnesic (Korsakoff) Syndrome. This syndrome is due to occlusion of the penetrating branches of the PCA that supply the midline areas of the thalamus. In this syndrome, memory is impaired to a much greater degree than other aspects of thought and behavior.

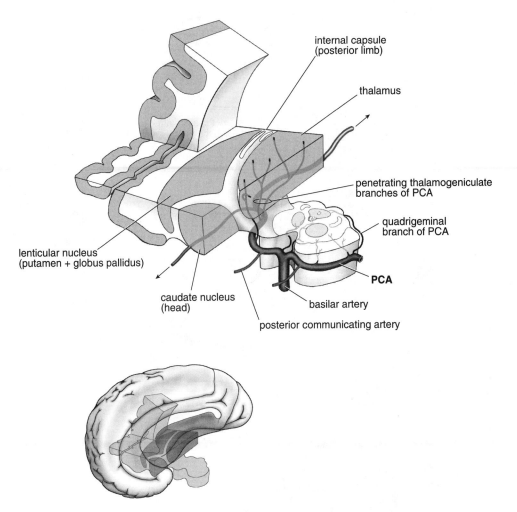

Figure 4-28. The penetrating branches of the posterior cerebral artery supply the thalamus (thalamogeniculate branches) and rostral portion of the midbrain. The right half of the brain and the entire midbrain are shown. Abbreviation: PCA, posterior cerebral artery.

- In a patient with Korsakoff's Syndrome, there is an impaired ability to recall events that had been well established before the occlusion (retrograde amnesia) as well as an impaired ability to learn or form new memories (anterograde amnesia).

Weber Syndrome (Paramedian Syndrome). This syndrome is also referred to as superior alternating hemiplegia. It is caused by infarction in the territory of the midbrain supplied by the paramedian penetrating branches of the PCA. These branches are sometimes called the interpeduncular branches (Figure 4-30A).

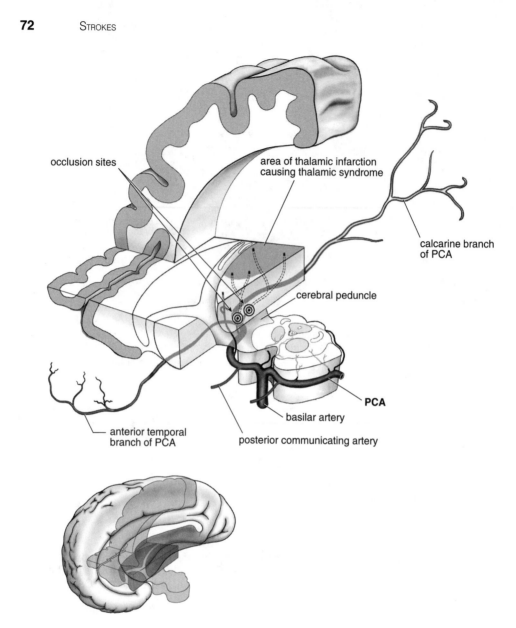

Figure 4-29. Occlusion of the thalamogeniculate branches of the posterior cerebral artery result in infarction of the thalamus producing the thalamic syndrome. The right half of the brain is shown. Abbreviation: PCA, posterior cerebral artery.

- There is a complete paralysis of specific muscles that move the eyes due to involvement of the third cranial nerve (the oculomotor nerve).
  - □ The deficits are referred to as an oculomotor nerve paralysis.
  - □ The eye on the side of the damage (the ipsilateral side) is deviated laterally (abducted) and depressed.

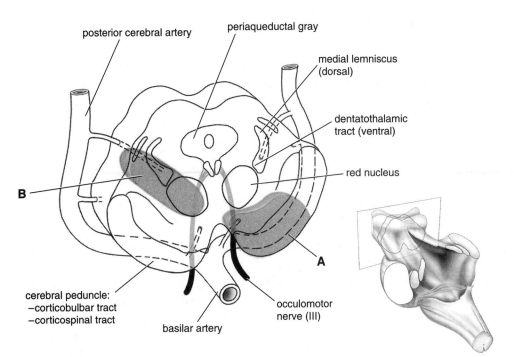

Figure 4-30. Transverse section through the rostral midbrain. The shaded areas show the primary regions infarcted when different penetrating branches of the PCA are occluded. A, with occlusion of the paramedian branches, Weber's Syndrome results. B, Benedikt's Syndrome results from occlusion of the penetrating branches that supply the tegmentum of the midbrain.

- □ The upper eyelid droops (ptosis).
- □ The pupil is dilated (mydriatic) and will not constrict properly when a light is shone in that eye (fixed pupil).
- • There is a weakness of the contralateral lower half of the face, tongue, and palate due to involvement of the corticobulbar tract in the cerebral peduncle.
- • There is a contralateral hemiparesis of the trunk and extremities due to involvement of the corticospinal tract, also running in the cerebral peduncle.

Benedikt Syndrome. This syndrome results from occlusion of penetrating branches of the PCA that supply the tegmentum of the midbrain (Figure 4-30B).

- • There is a complete oculomotor nerve paralysis (see Weber Syndrome).
- • There is an associated tremor in the contralateral extremities.
- • Movements of the extremities may also be uncoordinated (ataxic).
- • The tremor and ataxia are due to involvement of the dentatothalamic tract that connects the cerebellum with the thalamus.

Associated Signs. These deficits may occur in combination with symptoms characterizing the previous syndromes.

- Involvement of the thalamoperforant penetrating branches of the PCA commonly produce an extrapyramidal movement disorder called hemiballism.
  - Hemiballismus is due to infarction of the subthalamic nucleus.
  - The disorder consists of violent, forceful, flinging involuntary movements of the contralateral extremities.
- Infarction in the territory of the midbrain called the periaqueductal gray matter may result in so-called apathetic akinetic mutism.
  - The patient is in a drowsy, relatively immobile state from which she can be aroused only with strong stimulation.

Syndromes of the Cortical Branches. The various cortical branches of the PCA supply the inferior and medial parts of the temporal lobe and the medial surface of the occipital lobe. Figure 4-31 shows the cortical branches of the PCA. Figure 4-32 illustrates the functional areas of the cerebral cortex supplied by branches of the PCA. The medial portion of the temporal lobe is concerned with learning new information (re-

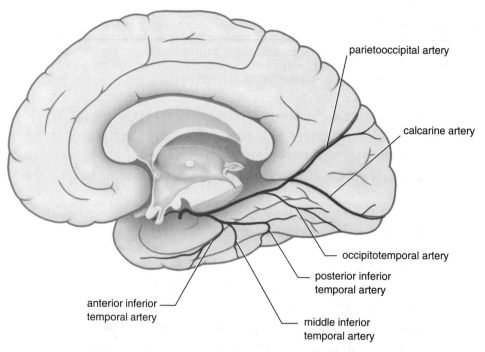

Figure 4-31. Medial surface of the right cerebral hemisphere. Cortical branches of the posterior cerebral artery supply the inferior and medial parts of the temporal lobe and the medial surface of the occipital lobe.

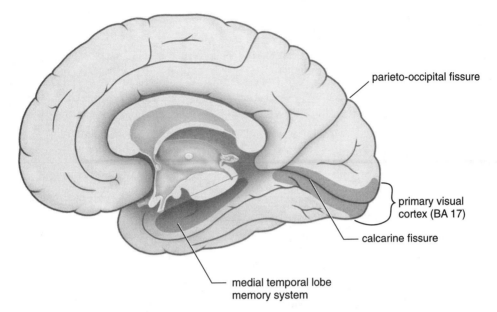

parieto-occipital fissure

primary visual cortex (BA 17)

calcarine fissure

medial temporal lobe memory system

Figure 4-32. Functional areas on the medial surface of the right hemisphere supplied by the posterior cerebral artery. The medial portion of the temporal lobe is concerned with recent memory. This includes the "submerged" cortex of the hippocampus. The medial portion of the occipital lobe is concerned with vision. Abbreviation: BA, Brodmann's area.

cent memory). The medial portion of the occipital lobe, supplied by the calcarine artery, is concerned with vision. Marked differences in symptoms occur when the occlusion involves just one side (unilateral) as opposed to occlusions that involve both sides (bilateral).

Syndromes of Unilateral Occlusion. Unilateral involvement of the calcarine branch of the PCA gives rise to a number of different signs.

- There may be a contralateral homonymous hemianopsia in which the patient loses vision in one-half of the visual field in *each* eye (hemianopsia) (Figure 4-33).

    □ The half field (hemi) of vision lost (anopsia) in each eye is the same (homonymous) and is in the visual field opposite (contralateral) to the side of the lesion. Hence the term *contralateral homonymous hemianopsia.*

    □ Central or macular vision may be spared because of collateral circulation to the portion of the occipital pole where the central portion of the retina is represented.

        ◆ This collateral circulation comes from the distal branches of the MCA or ACA.

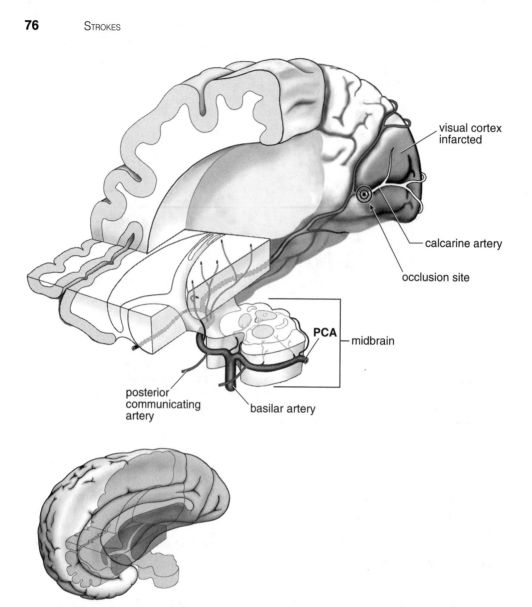

Figure 4-33. Occlusion affecting the calcarine branch of the posterior cerebral artery. Involvement of the calcarine branch leads to a contralateral homonymous hemianopsia. The right half of the brain is shown. Abbreviation: PCA, posterior cerebral artery.

- The syndrome of alexia without agraphia may occur with involvement of the PCA in the dominant hemisphere.

  □ The person loses the ability to read aloud and to understand written language (alexia).

    ♦ Amazingly, the patient retains the ability to write spontaneously (does not have agraphia), but then cannot read what has just been written.

  □ The patient may be unable to name objects or to match a seen color with its spoken name.

- The lesion causing alexia without agraphia destroys the left visual cortex and underlying geniculocalcarine tract as well as the fibers of the corpus callosum that connect the intact right visual cortex with the intact language areas of the dominant left hemisphere (Figure 4-34).

  □ As a consequence of the left occipital lesion, the patient is blind in the right half of each visual field so that written visual information reaches only the right occipital lobe.

  □ In order to be read (as language), words perceived in the right visual cortex must cross over to the language area of the left hemisphere.

    ◆ The lesion to the fibers of the corpus callosum prevents this transfer of written visual information from occurring, hence the alexia.

Syndromes of Bilateral Occlusion. Bilateral infarctions may cause signs and symptoms quite different than those associated with unilateral infarctions. Bilateral infarctions of the occipital lobes can produce a variety of deficits (Figure 4-35):

- When extensive, bilateral occipital lobe lesions result in total blindness (cortical blindness), that is, a bilateral homonymous hemianopsia.

  □ Occasionally, Anton's Syndrome results.

    ◆ The patient is unaware of being blind and may collide with objects when attempting to walk.

    ◆ The patient may even deny being blind when it is pointed out.

- More often, the bilateral infarctions are less extensive and portions of the visual field remain intact.

- When the occipital poles are spared, the patient has central ("gun barrel") vision.

- In contrast, when the occipital poles alone are infarcted there is a selective loss of central vision only.

- The Balint Syndrome is another possible consequence of bilateral occipital lesions. The Balint Syndrome consists of:

  □ The patient cannot voluntarily look into the peripheral field of vision, even though there is no paralysis of the muscles that move the eyeballs.

  □ Optic ataxia, which expresses itself as the patient's failure to grasp or touch an object when the movement is guided by vision.

    ◆ To reach an object placed on a tabletop, the patient searches for the object by running his hand along the tabletop.

  □ Visual inattention, which expresses itself by the patient being unable to find a series of objects or a failure to connect a series of dots by lines.

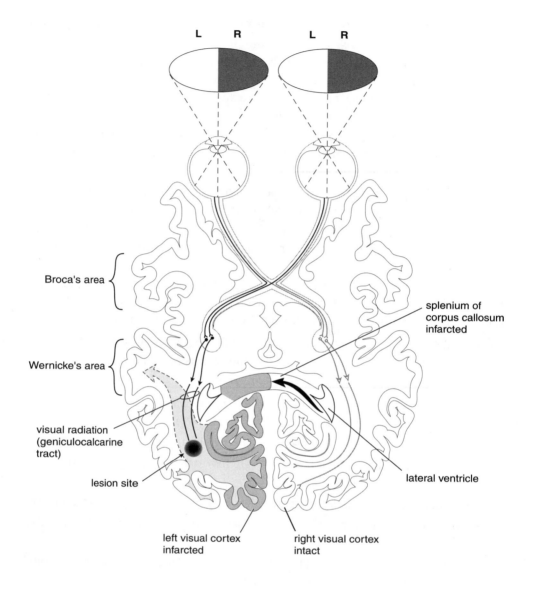

Broca's area

splenium of
corpus callosum
infarcted

Wernicke's area

visual radiation
(geniculocalcarine
tract)

lesion site

lateral ventricle

left visual cortex
infarcted

right visual cortex
intact

FIGURE 4-34. Horizontal section through the cerebral hemispheres. The visual fields are shown in front of the retina to indicate the patient is blind in the right half field of vision in each eye (i.e., a right homonymous hemianopsia). This visual deficit is caused by a lesion in the left occipital white matter at the indicated site. The lesion destroys the left visual radiation and also prevents information from the intact right visual cortex from reaching Wernicke's area in the left hemisphere. Thus, the patient cannot read (alexia) words that are "seen" by the right visual cortex. However, the patient can still speak (no aphasia) and write (no agraphia). Infarctions in the splenium of the corpus callosum and left visual cortex (shaded) would have a similar effect.

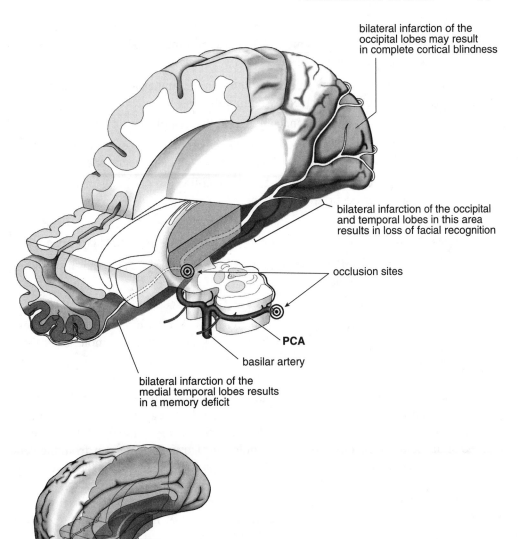

bilateral infarction of the
occipital lobes may result
in complete cortical blindness

bilateral infarction of the occipital
and temporal lobes in this area
results in loss of facial recognition

occlusion sites

PCA

basilar artery

bilateral infarction of the
medial temporal lobes results
in a memory deficit

Figure 4-35.   Areas of the occipital and temporal lobes infarcted with occlusion of the posterior cerebral artery. For clarity, only the right hemisphere is shown but similar cortical areas in the left hemisphere also would be damaged. The deficits resulting from bilateral occlusion of the posterior cerebral artery are quite different from those resulting from blockage of the artery on just one side. See text. The right half of the brain and the entire midbrain are shown. Abbreviation: PCA, posterior cerebral artery.

Bilateral lesions of the inferior and medial parts of the temporal lobe may result in a Korsakoff Syndrome. (Remember that this syndrome can also occur with occlusion of the penetrating branches of the PCA.)

- In addition to the retrograde and anterograde amnesia, the Korsakoff Syndrome may be characterized by confabulation.
  - Confabulation is the inaccurate recollection of memories.
  - It may take the form of partially remembered experiences that are recalled without regard to their actual sequence of occurrence.
  - More rarely, it may consist of the recollection of events or experiences that never occurred (fantasies).

Bilateral lesions involving the ventral and medial region of the occipital and temporal lobes may result in a lack of recognition of faces, a disorder called prosopagnosia.

- The patient cannot identify a familiar face, even a spouse, either by looking at the person or a picture.
- The patient knows that a face is a face and can point out individual facial features.
- In order to identify a person, the patient has to rely on the sound of the person's voice, or on a specific facial feature such as glasses, a mole, or beard.

The Vertebral Artery

In visualizing the blood supply of the brain stem and the stroke syndromes resulting from its infarction, we have adopted the same general strategy as used with the brain. Figure 4-36 presents the overall pattern of the arterial supply to the three subdivisions of the brain stem: the medulla, pons, and midbrain. This supply derives from the vertebrobasilar system. (Figure 4-27 shows the vertebrobasilar supply of the brain stem from a lateral perspective.) Subsequent figures, for example Figure 4-37, isolate a single cross-section from a particular level of the brain stem (shown in the inset to each figure). The specific structures residing in that section of the brain stem are shown along with their arterial supply. The set of structures damaged when a particular vessel is occluded is indicated by shading.

Two vertebral arteries, one on each side, enter the cranium and course along the ventral surface of the medulla (Figures 4-27, 4-36). Each artery passes upward and medially, and the two vertebral arteries join at the lower border of the pons to form the single basilar artery. On each side, the intracranial branches of the vertebral arteries are the posterior spinal artery, the posterior inferior cerebellar artery, the anterior spinal artery, and the bulbar branches.

The vertebral arteries are the main arteries supplying the medulla, the most inferior division of the brain stem, which is continuous with the spinal cord. However, the relative sizes of the vertebral arteries and their branches vary considerably. In addition, there may be considerable overlap in the areas supplied by some vessels. As a result, the neurological deficits produced by vertebral artery occlusion can be quite variable.

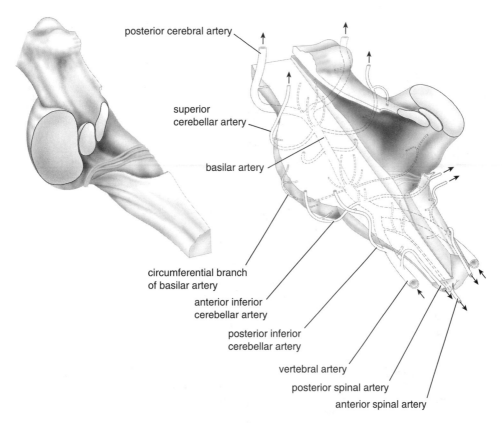

posterior cerebral artery

superior cerebellar artery

basilar artery

circumferential branch of basilar artery

anterior inferior cerebellar artery

posterior inferior cerebellar artery

vertebral artery

posterior spinal artery

anterior spinal artery

Figure 4-36. The brain stem is viewed from behind with the cerebellum removed. The left dorsal one-third of the brain stem has been cut away so we can visualize the general organization of the vertebral-basilar arterial system supplying the brain stem. Not all branches are shown and there is considerable variability in the sizes of the vessels as well as overlap in the areas supplied by some vessels.

Lateral Medullary Syndrome (Wallenberg's Syndrome). This is the most common vascular syndrome of the entire brain stem. It can occur in either a complete or modified form. Wallenberg's Syndrome is most often attributed to occlusion of the posterior inferior cerebellar artery. However, because of the variability of the brain stem's blood supply it is incorrect to regard Wallenberg's Syndrome as synonymous with posterior inferior cerebellar artery occlusion. Most cases actually may be due to occlusion of the parent vertebral artery. In either situation, a wedge-shaped region of the lateral medulla is infarcted (Figure 4-37B). The full-blown Wallenberg Syndrome includes:

- Impairment of pain and temperature sense over the contralateral (opposite to the side of the infarct) half of the body due to involvement of the spinothalamic tract.

- Loss of pain and temperature sensation over all or part of the ipsilateral half of the face due to involvement of the spinal trigeminal system.

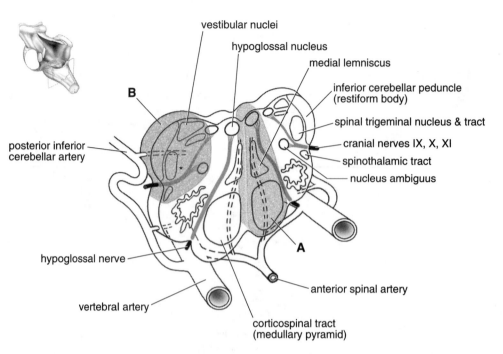

vestibular nuclei

hypoglossal nucleus

medial lemniscus

inferior cerebellar peduncle
(restiform body)

B

spinal trigeminal nucleus & tract

cranial nerves IX, X, XI

posterior inferior
cerebellar artery

spinothalamic tract

nucleus ambiguus

A

hypoglossal nerve

anterior spinal artery

vertebral artery

corticospinal tract
(medullary pyramid)

Figure 4-37. Transverse section through the medulla showing the areas damaged (shaded). In A, the medial medullary syndrome (rare) and in B, the more common complete Wallenberg Syndrome (also called the lateral medullary syndrome).
* indicates the area of the descending sympathetic tract that, when damaged, produces a Horner's Syndrome.

    □ There also may be pain in the face.

- An ipsilateral Horner's Syndrome due to involvement of the descending sympathetic tract.

    □ A small pupil (meiosis).

    □ Drooping of the upper eyelid (ptosis).

    □ Decreased sweating on one side of the face (anhydrosis).

- A number of signs and symptoms are due to involvement of the nucleus ambiguus and fibers of cranial nerves IX, X, and XI.

    □ Hoarseness (dysphonia).

    □ Difficulty swallowing (dysphagia).

    □ Difficulty speaking (dysarthria).

    □ Diminished gag reflex.

    □ Hiccups.

- A variety of signs and symptoms are due to involvement of the vestibular nuclei.

    □ Involuntary rhythmic movements of the eyes (nystagmus).

- □ Double vision (diplopia).
- □ The sensation that objects are oscillating when looking at them (oscillopsia).
- □ The sensation that the patient is turning or that external objects are whirling (vertigo).
- □ Nausea and vomiting.
- □ Lateropulsion, the tendency to fall sideways (ipsiversive) without accompanying vertigo.
- Ipsilateral incoordination of movements (ataxia) due to involvement of fibers projecting to the cerebellum (olivocerebellar, spinocerebellar, and/or inferior cerebellar peduncle).

Medial (Paramedial) Medullary Syndrome. This rare syndrome results from occlusion of the anterior spinal artery. The resultant infarction is in a vertical strip of brain stem tissue adjacent to the midline of the medulla (Figure 4-37A). The syndrome is also called inferior alternating hemiplegia. The syndrome is characterized by:

- Paralysis and atrophy of the ipsilateral one-half of the tongue due to involvement of the fibers of the XIIth (hypoglossal) cranial nerve.
- Spastic paralysis of the contralateral arm and leg due to involvement of the medullary pyramid containing fibers of the corticospinal tract.
- Loss or impairment in position, vibration, and discriminative touch sensations on the contralateral one-half of the body due to involvement of sensory axons in the medial lemniscus.

The Basilar Artery

The pons is supplied by branches of the basilar artery as is much of the cerebellum (Figure 4-36). Vascular lesions of the pons result in a number of different syndromes.

Medial (Paramedian) Inferior Pontine Syndrome. This syndrome, also called middle alternating hemiplegia, results from occlusion of the paramedian branches of the basilar artery, which supply a wedge of pons on either side of the midline (Figure 4-38A). Occlusion of these branches on one side produces the following symptoms and signs:

- Medial deviation of the ipsilateral eye due to a weakness of the lateral rectus muscle from infarction of the fibers of the VIth (abducens) cranial nerve.
  - □ This also causes double vision when looking to the side.
- Inability to look laterally toward the side of the lesion (paralysis of conjugate gaze) due to involvement of the pontine center for lateral gaze.
- Contralateral spastic paralysis of the lower face, arm, and leg due to involvement of the pyramidal tract (consisting of the corticospinal and corticobulbar tracts).

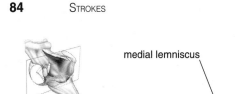

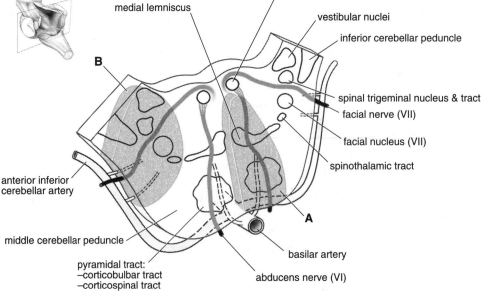

Figure 4-38. Transverse section through the inferior pons. A, area damaged (shaded) in the medial inferior pontine syndrome. B, area damaged (shaded) in the lateral inferior pontine syndrome (also called syndrome of the anterior inferior cerebellar artery).

- Impaired tactile (touch), vibration, and proprioceptive (position) sensation on the opposite half of the body due to involvement of the medial lemniscus.

- Uncoordinated movements of the limbs and gait (ataxia) due to involvement of fibers projecting to the cerebellum (these axons run in the middle cerebellar peduncle).

Lateral Inferior Pontine Syndrome (Syndrome of the Anterior Inferior Cerebellar Artery). This syndrome results from occlusion of the anterior inferior cerebellar artery, which supplies the lateral two-thirds of the pons and the anterior and inferior portion of the cerebellum (Figure 4-38B). The following neurological deficits may be seen:

- Paralysis of the muscles of the entire ipsilateral one-half of the face due to involvement of the facial nucleus or nerve (VIIth cranial nerve).

- Absent taste sensation over the anterior two-thirds of the tongue on the side of the lesion due to involvement of the facial nerve or solitary nucleus.

- Inability to close the ipsilateral eye when it is touched with a wisp of cotton (loss of the corneal reflex) due to involvement of the facial nucleus or nerve.

- Deafness on the side of the lesion due to involvement of the cochlear nuclei or nerve (part of the VIIIth cranial nerve).

- Nystagmus, vertigo, nausea, vomiting, and oscillopsia due to involvement of the vestibular nuclei or nerve (part of the VIIIth cranial nerve).

- Ipsilateral loss of pain and temperature sensation from the face due to involvement of the spinal trigeminal nucleus and tract.

- Uncoordinated movements (ataxia) of the limbs and gait on the side of the lesion due to involvement of fibers projecting to the cerebellum (these axons run in the middle and inferior cerebellar peduncles).

- Impaired pain and temperature sense over half the body on the contralateral side due to involvement of the spinothalamic tract.

- Ipsilateral Horner's Syndrome due to involvement of the descending sympathetic tract.

  ▫ Meiosis

  ▫ Ptosis

  ▫ Anhydrosis of one-half the face

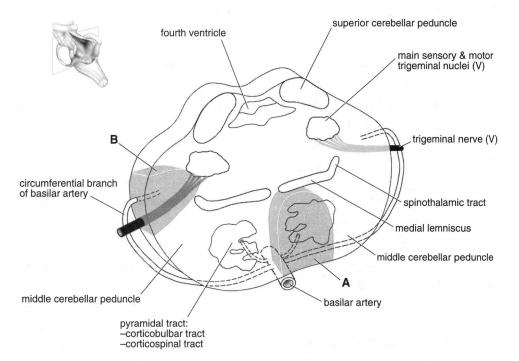

Figure 4-39. Transverse section through the middle of the pons. A, area damaged (shaded) in the medial midpontine syndrome. B, area damaged (shaded) in the lateral midpontine syndrome.

Medial Midpontine Syndrome. This syndrome results from occlusion of the paramedian branches originating from the middle portion of the basilar artery (Figure 4-39A). The syndrome is usually a purely motor syndrome.

- Ataxia of the limbs and gait on the side of the lesion due to involvement of fibers projecting to the cerebellum (middle cerebellar peduncle).
- Paralysis of the arm, leg, and lower half of the face on the side opposite the lesion due to involvement of the pyramidal tract (corticobulbar and corticospinal tracts).

Lateral Midpontine Syndrome. This syndrome results from occlusion of the short circumferential branch of the basilar artery supplying the lateral two-thirds of the pons (Figure 4-39B).

- Ataxia of the limbs on the side of the lesion due to involvement of fibers projecting to the cerebellum (middle cerebellar peduncle).
- A number of signs are due to involvement of the trigeminal nerve or nucleus:
  - Ipsilateral paralysis of the muscles of mastication.
  - Deviation of the jaw to the side of the lesion.
  - Impaired sensation over the side of the face on the side of the lesion.
  - Loss of the corneal reflex.

Medial (Paramedian) Superior Pontine Syndrome. This syndrome results from occlusion of the paramedian branches (Figure 4-40A). The syndrome is usually a purely motor syndrome.

- Ataxia of the limbs and gait on the side of the lesion due to involvement of fibers projecting to the cerebellum (middle cerebellar peduncle).
- Paralysis of the arm, leg, and lower half of the face on the side opposite the lesion due to involvement of the corticospinal and corticobulbar tracts.
- Impaired tactile (touch), vibration, and proprioceptive (position) sensation on the opposite half of the body due to involvement of the medial lemniscus occurs infrequently.

Lateral Superior Pontine Syndrome (Syndrome of the Superior Cerebellar Artery). This syndrome results from occlusion of the superior cerebellar artery, the last long circumferential branch of the basilar artery (Figure 4-40B). It supplies the lateral pons and cerebellum.

- Ataxia of the limbs and gait on the side of the lesion, falling to the side of the lesion, and intention tremor on the side of the lesion due to involvement of fibers projecting to or coming from the cerebellum (middle and superior cerebellar peduncles) and to involvement of the cerebellum itself.

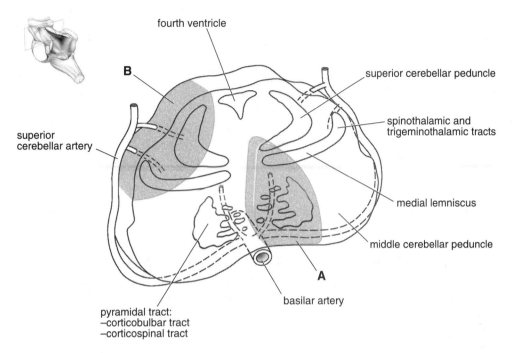

fourth ventricle

B

superior cerebellar peduncle

superior
cerebellar artery

spinothalamic and
trigeminothalamic tracts

medial lemniscus

middle cerebellar peduncle

A

basilar artery

pyramidal tract:
–corticobulbar tract
–corticospinal tract

Figure 4-40. Transverse section through the superior pons. A, area damaged (shaded) in the medial superior pontine syndrome. B, area damaged (shaded) in the lateral superior pontine syndrome (also called syndrome of the superior cerebellar artery).

- Contralateral loss of pain and temperature sensation from the trunk, leg, arm, and face due to involvement of the spinothalamic and trigeminothalamic (face) tracts.

- Contralateral loss of discriminative touch, vibration, and position sense more in the leg than in the arm due to involvement of the medial lemniscus.

- Ipsilateral Horner's Syndrome due to involvement of the descending sympathetic tract:

  □ Meiosis

  □ Ptosis

  □ Anhydrosis of one-half the face

Complete Basilar Syndrome. This syndrome results from bilateral occlusion that affects both paramedian and circumferential arteries. Such bilateral occlusion produces an incomplete ischemic transection of the brain stem.

- Usually the patient is in a coma and shows pinpoint, irregular, or unequal pupils, bilateral conjugate gaze paralysis, or internuclear opthalmoplegia, and paralysis of all limbs. Few of these patients survive for more than a few days.

Locked-in Syndrome. Although rare, this syndrome also may follow occlusion of the basilar artery. But it is quite distinct from syndromes in which consciousness is disturbed, as in the complete basilar syndrome discussed in which coma occurs. An infarct confined to the ventral pons spares both the ascending somatosensory pathways responsible for the perception of bodily sensations, as well as the ascending system of neurons that is responsible for maintaining arousal and wakefulness. As a result, the patient is conscious—he is alert, aware of his environment, understands what is said to him, etc. However, the lesion interrupts the corticospinal and corticobulbar tracts located in the ventral pons leaving the patient in a state of near total motor paralysis including an inability to speak and eat. Thus, although consciousness is retained, it is virtually inexpressible. In the full-blown locked-in syndrome, only eye opening, vertical (not lateral) eye movements, and convergence remain.

None of us is likely to relate, even remotely, to the experience of enduring what certainly must be the ultimate in agonizing frustration. However, the late Jean-Dominique Bauby, in an autobiography painstakingly put to paper by an assistant transcribing Bauby's eye blinks, describes his "locked-in experience" in *The Diving Bell and the Butterfly.*

TREATMENT

It is unusual for a patient who has suffered a stroke to be brought to medical attention within minutes of the stroke onset. Generally, several hours will have elapsed before a diagnosis is made. According to some reports an average of about 6 hours will have elapsed between stroke onset and diagnosis. During this time the stroke may continue to evolve and worsen (a stroke in evolution). Unfortunately, once ischemia has occurred (even if the stroke does not increase in severity), it sets into motion a cascade of cellular events resulting in the destruction of increasing numbers of nerve cells in areas of brain tissue surrounding the initial ischemic event. This area of vulnerability surrounding the initial zone of ischemia is called the penumbra. No available (approved by the FDA) treatment is able to interrupt any step in this cascade to slow or prevent nerve cell death in the penumbra.

Patients who have suffered a major stroke as a result of ischemic infarction (the vast majority of stroke patients) are kept horizontal in bed for the first few days. This is because assuming an upright posture may cause a decrease in cerebral circulation and thus aggravate ischemia. Medical management focuses on maintaining normal blood pressure.

When the common or internal carotid artery has just become occluded, surgical removal of the clot or a surgical bypass procedure may be carried out. However, after a period of 12 hours the opening of an occluded vessel is of no benefit. Once ischemic neurologic damage has occurred, no currently available treatment has conclusively been demonstrated to favorably influence the outcome of the brain injury.

Treatment of Cerebral Edema

Some degree of edema surrounds all cerebral infarcts. Brain cells themselves take in increased amounts of water. In addition, excess water is drawn into the extracellular space surrounding brain cells. Edema becomes detectable within 12 to 24 hours following infarction and may continue to increase for another 48 hours.

Following massive cerebral infarction, cerebral edema may be life-threatening. This is because large edematous cerebral infarcts can cause a herniation of brain tissue (Figure 4-4). Specific herniations can compress those portions of the brain stem controlling respiration, heart rate, and blood pressure. When brain herniation threatens, intravenous dehydrating agents such as mannitol may be given in an effort to shrink the brain. Passive hyperventilation may reduce intracranial pressure by causing arterial vasoconstriction for 1 or 2 hours. The practice of inducing a coma by the administration of an anesthetic greatly complicates patient care and has no proven therapeutic value. Corticosteroid drugs are not administered because they may cause hyperglycemia, which risks worsening the stroke.

Anticoagulant Drugs

Once a stroke is fully developed, the administration of anticoagulants is of no value. The use of anticoagulants in acute stroke is controversial because of the associated risk of hemorrhage that approaches 20 percent with a mortality of 1 percent.

Intravenous heparin therapy is initiated at the time of hospital admission in certain patients. Such patients fall into one of the following categories: (1) Those experiencing repetitive, closely spaced transient ischemic attacks; (2) those with a progression of signs such as weakness in the hours before hospitalization; (3) those observed to have increasing neurologic deficits in the first 18 hours after admission; and (4) those demonstrating fluctuating neurologic signs and symptoms of vertebral, basilar, or carotid ischemia. Before anticoagulant therapy is initiated, a CT scan is obtained to rule out hemorrhage. Heparin therapy may be maintained for up to two weeks.

Heparin therapy may be replaced gradually with oral warfarin, which is the most effective of the coumarin derivatives. Warfarin replacement therapy is instituted in patients whose evolving stroke halted when they received heparin and in those patients who have a high risk for future embolization such as those with atrial fibrillation.

Warfarin therapy can continue out of hospital for months or years *when* adequate supervision can be guaranteed, but the trend now is not to give warfarin indefinitely. The greatest usefulness of warfarin is in the first two to four months after the onset of ischemic strokes. With the long-term administration of anticoagulant, the risk of hemorrhage outweighs the benefit from prevention of stroke. For example, the risk of intracerebral hemorrhage or subdural hematoma in patients over 50 years of age taking an oral anticoagulant over a long term may be increased tenfold.

Antiplatelet Drugs

Several large clinical trials have suggested that aspirin (80mg to 1.5gms daily) given to persons experiencing TIAs or with coronary artery disease reduces the risk of recurrent cerebral TIAs and thrombotic and embolic strokes. However, a significant number of patients still experience ischemic strokes while receiving aspirin. Aspirin acts to inhibit platelet aggregation.

When aspirin cannot be tolerated, the platelet aggregate inhibitor ticlopidine (TICLID) may be used. It has not been established that other antiaggregant drugs such as dipyridamole (PERSANTINE) and sulfinpyrazone (ANTURANE) are of benefit. Platelet antiaggregants are frequently used as a preventative measure to treat patients considered at high risk for stroke. Platelet antiaggregants also are administered to patients experiencing infrequent carotid or vertebrobasilar TIAs, and are used for the chronic treatment of patients who have had a completed stroke.

Thrombolytic Agents

Thrombolytic agents are drugs that break up or dissolve a thrombus. The formation of a blood clot (thrombus) is a natural response to blood vessel injury. A blood protein called fibrin is involved in the formation of a blood clot. However, a clot does not represent a permanent solution to blood vessel injury. Thus, once vessel healing has occurred, a process called fibrinolysis removes unneeded clots. Without this naturally occurring fibrinolysis, blood vessels would gradually become completely occluded by the progressive accumulation of unremoved clots. The naturally occurring clot dissolver is a fibrin-digesting enzyme called plasmin. Plasmin is produced when a blood protein called plasminogen is activated. Large amounts of plasminogen exist within a thrombus, but it remains inactive until a specific signal reaches it. The appropriate signal is called tissue plasminogen activator (t-PA). The presence of a clot causes t-PA to be secreted by the endothelial cells forming the blood vessel wall. Tissue plasminogen activator activates plasminogen, which produces the plasmin that dissolves the clot. Most plasminogen occurs within the clot itself so that plasmin activity is largely confined to the clot.

Tissue-type plasminogen activator (t-PA) has been approved by the FDA as a therapy for acute ischemic stroke. In the study used by the FDA to support its approval of t-PA, 31 percent of patients with acute ischemic stroke treated with t-PA had an excellent outcome at three months compared with 20 percent of patients treated with a placebo. The major risk of t-PA treatment is that it may cause intracerebral hemorrhage. When this risk is included, the correct question to ask patients is whether they would risk an 11 percent chance of an improved neurological outcome following ischemic stroke against a 3 percent chance of early death from t-PA-induced intracerebral hemorrhage. It is important to emphasize that patients with the most severe neurological deficits, and, therefore, those most likely to gain from t-PA treatment, are the very patients most at risk to develop intracerebral hemorrhage.

If patients with ischemic stroke are to be treated successfully with t-PA, they must be treated in the same way those in the approval study just mentioned were treated. Thus, patients must be treated with t-PA within hours of symptom onset. Treatment of patients after 3 hours with t-PA may be dangerous. Once treatment is initiated, patients must be carefully monitored to avoid hypertension and in order for the physician to be able to promptly detect signs and symptoms of intracerebral hemorrhage. Patients in the FDA study were carefully selected. It is questionable whether this level of efficiency could be duplicated easily in routine clinical practice.

Surgery

Before surgery is performed, the presence, location, and extent of the lesion must be determined with arteriography (angiography). Arteriography involves the injection of a radiopaque contrast medium into arteries in order to visualize them by x-ray imaging. Arteriography carries a risk of 1 to 2 percent of causing serious complications by worsening the stroke or producing focal neurologic deficits.

Surgical therapy is attempted only in those patients with internal carotid artery stenosis and ulcerated plaques located in the neck. The surgical procedure is called carotid endarterectomy. The procedure involves excision of the occluding atheromatous deposits so as to leave a smooth arterial lining. In patients with a greater than 80 percent occlusion of the internal carotid artery the procedure is effective in preventing ipsilateral cerebral strokes.

Rehabilitation Therapy

A sometimes considered general guideline is that patients whose neurological deficits do not improve completely within two to three weeks will benefit from an organized program of physical therapy. The time to initiate therapy, however, need not be delayed for this length of time. Therapy may be started as soon as the patient has stabilized medically. Thus, in appropriate patients, therapy may be initiated within a day of admission to a hospital.

Prevention of contracture is important and can be accomplished by passively moving paralyzed limbs through a full range of motion many times a day. Many hemiplegics regain at least some ability to walk within three to six months. A major limiting factor in regaining the ability to walk is the presence of a proprioceptive sensory loss. The patient with such a loss, without using vision, is unable to recognize the occurrence of muscle contractions, the position of the limbs in space, or whether the limbs are moving or stationary. In the absence of this proprioceptive and visual information, the parts of the brain that control movement cannot do so effectively.

Speech therapy may be initiated in appropriate patients. Speech therapists can provide valuable insights in patient assessment and help design compensating communication strategies. They can play an important role in the management of dysarthria. Therapists also can help manage dysphagia, which may be a common problem in the acute stage of recovery. The degree to which therapy improves aphasic symptomatology beyond the benefit resulting from the intervention of human-to-human contact is uncertain. But clearly, improving the patient's morale with such contact can spur the motivation to recover.

In alert and responsive patients whose motor function has improved, occupational therapy may be undertaken. This therapy instructs the patient in the activities of daily living and in the use of special devices that can assist the patient in becoming independent.

Chapter 5

EMBOLIC INFARCTION

Cerebral embolism may result from a variety of disorders, but it usually is a result of cardiovascular disease. Indeed, it is essentially a manifestation of heart disease. Fully 75 percent of cardiac emboli lodge in the brain. Generally, the embolic material consists of a fragment that has broken away from a thrombus within the heart. Less often, the embolus is a fragment from an atherosclerotic plaque that has ulcerated into the lumen of an artery (Figure 4-3D). Following trauma, embolization of fat or air may occur but this is rare. Emboli composed of tumor cells also are rare.

The development of a thrombus in the heart is most commonly the result of chronic atrial fibrillation due to atherosclerotic or rheumatic heart disease. The rapid and irregular contractions (fibrillation) of heart muscle result in the development of a clot in the left atrium because blood no longer flows smoothly through the heart. This is called a mural thrombus. A mural thrombus may also form on the damaged endocardium (inner lining of the heart) overlying an area of myocardial infarction. Sudden changes in cardiac rhythm, such as occurs when the fibrillating heart returns to a normal rhythm, may result in the breaking off of a fragment of thrombotic material which then enters the circulation as an embolus.

Embolic material will travel in the circulation until it reaches a vessel whose lumen is too small to permit further passage of the embolus (Figure 5-1). Once lodged in a vessel, the embolus may remain and plug the lumen solidly. More often, however, the embolus breaks into smaller fragments which then enter smaller vessels, sometimes to disappear entirely.

The infarct resulting from an embolic stroke may be pale, hemorrhagic, or mixed. Most embolic infarcts are pale. However, the development of secondary hemorrhage into an area of pale embolic infarction does occur. This is due to the breaking up of the embolic material that has been blocking an artery. With the passage of the embolic material into more distal branches of the vessel, the necrotic area again receives blood under normal pressure. However, being in the area of necrosis, the walls of arteries also have been ischemic and thus have been damaged. As a result, when again perfused

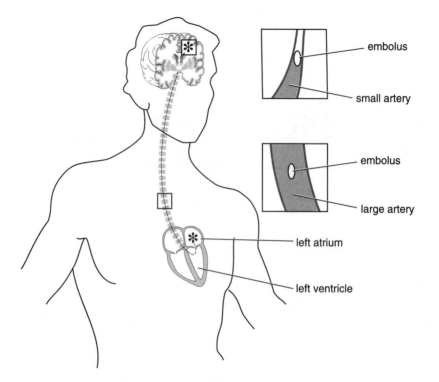

embolus

small artery

embolus

large artery

left atrium

left ventricle

Figure 5-1. Cerebral embolism most commonly results from embolic material that originated in the heart. Heart disease sometimes leads to the development of a thrombus ("clot") in the chambers of the heart. A fragment of the thrombus can break off to form an embolus. The embolus then travels in the arterial system until it reaches an artery in the brain whose diameter is too small for the embolus to travel any further. By blocking the artery, blood cannot reach brain tissue distal to the embolus, resulting in infarction of the blood-starved tissue.

under a normal head of pressure, the damaged arterial wall leaks and blood escapes into the surrounding necrotic brain tissue.

Hemorrhagic infarcts occur in about 30 percent of cases. Evidence of this hemorrhage may appear in the cerebrospinal fluid (CSF) as red blood cells or a discoloration of CSF produced by products resulting from the breakdown of red blood cells (xanthocromia). The appearance of RBCs in the CSF occurs only in a minority of cases of hemorrhagic infarct due to embolism.

CLINICAL COURSE AND PROGNOSIS

A number of factors are important in differentiating embolic from atherothrombotic infarction. Most important is the suddenness with which an embolic stroke develops. The full-blown set of deficits evolves within several seconds or a minute with embolic occlusion. The event may be so sudden that the patient stops speaking in mid-sentence with a total loss of speech. With atherothrombotic strokes, the clinical picture evolves over hours or longer. Second, embolic strokes usually are not accompanied by warning events such as TIAs. In contrast, atherothrombotic strokes are often preceded by one or more TIAs. Third, embolic occlusions may occur during any time of the day and often occur during periods of activity. Atherothrombotic infarctions tend to occur during sleep. Fourth, recurrent convulsive seizures are more likely to occur with embolic cortical infarcts and are uncommon consequences of thrombotic strokes. Fifth, infarction resulting from embolic occlusion is more likely to be hemorrhagic than is infarction from atherothrombotic occlusion. Finally, embolic occlusions often produce neurologic deficits, even severe deficits, that are only temporary. With disintegration of the embolic material blood flow is restored and signs and symptoms disappear.

STROKE SYNDROMES

Multiple small emboli may occur over a period of months or years and result in a dementia in addition to focal neurologic deficits. Such cases are referred to as multi-infarct dementia. Patients with multi-infarct dementia also have emboli that involve structures other than the brain such as the kidney, spleen, and skin. Emboli involving the kidney often can be detected by the appearance of red blood cells in the urine (hematuria).

Single larger emboli result in a neurologic picture that varies with the vessel involved and the location of the embolus. In the internal carotid system, such emboli occlude vessels and cause signs and symptoms that are the same as those outlined under stroke syndromes in Chapter 4. In some cases, a single large embolus will occlude the internal carotid artery or the stem of the MCA resulting in the complete clinical picture occurring with occlusion of the particular vessel. More often, however, the embolus is smaller and occludes branches of the MCA, particularly the left MCA. Such branch occlusion can produce a very focal disorder such as a Broca's aphasia or a Wernicke's aphasia with little or no paralysis.

In the vertebral-basilar system, an embolus most often will pass through the vertebral artery and the larger basilar artery and will not lodge until it reaches the bifurcation of the basilar artery. When it lodges at this location, it may produce deep coma and total paralysis. More often, however, the embolus will continue into one or both PCAs and result in infarction of one or both visual cortices. This produces a unilateral or bilateral homonymous hemianopsia.

Most patients survive the initial embolic infarct and the long-term prognosis is then determined by several factors. One is the occurrence of additional embolization which happens in about 80 percent of patients. There is no basis for predicting when this may occur. Another factor is the severity of the underlying disease (e.g., cardiac failure, myocardial infarction, endocarditis) that caused embolization.

TREATMENT

The treatment of cerebral emboli involves the prevention of additional embolic episodes. In cases of atrial fibrillation and myocardial infarction, the long-term use (two years) of anticoagulants such as warfarin significantly reduces the incidence of recurrent strokes.

Once embolization has occurred, management during the acute phase may be difficult. The administration of anticoagulants is initiated once it has been determined that the infarct is not hemorrhagic. Otherwise, there is a risk of additional bleeding into the infarct. It may require time for a hemorrhagic infarct to become apparent on a CT scan. In patients who have sustained a large infarct and are hypertensive, anticoagulant therapy is avoided in the acute phase. In cases where it has been determined that the infarct is not hemorrhagic, intravenous heparin is followed by warfarin.

Chapter 6

CEREBRAL HEMORRHAGE

Spontaneous (nontraumatic) hemorrhage is the third most common cause of stroke, following atherothrombosis and embolism. Our concern in this chapter is with hemorrhage that occurs primarily into the substance of the brain. These are called intracerebral, or parenchymal hemorrhages. About 90 percent of spontaneous intracerebral hemorrhages occur when a brain-penetrating artery is damaged and finally ruptures due to hypertension and atherosclerosis. Blood escapes from the ruptured vessel (extravasates) and forms a roughly circular or oval mass that destroys brain tissue and grows in volume as the bleeding continues. In patients with hypertension, the occurrence of bleeding tends to parallel the intensity and duration of hypertension.

The extravasated mass of blood displaces and compresses adjacent brain tissue. When large (several centimeters in diameter), the hemorrhage may displace midline brain stem structures thereby compromising vital centers and lead to coma and death (Figure 6-1). Large hemorrhages also usually result in blood leaking into the ventricular system thereby causing the cerebrospinal fluid (CSF) to become bloody. In contrast, CSF remains clear with small hemorrhages that are located at a distance from the brain ventricles.

CLINICAL COURSE AND PROGNOSIS

Most primary intracerebral hemorrhages begin during wakefulness and activity in contrast to ischemic strokes, which begin during sleep. Blacks are affected more often than whites. A sudden severe headache ("the worst of my life") usually occurs just before the onset of the stroke, but is absent or mild in degree in many cases.

Nausea and vomiting at the onset of a hemorrhagic stroke occurs much more often than with ischemic strokes. In about 10 percent of patients, focal cerebral seizures occur. Drowsiness, confusion, loss of consciousness, and periodic increases in the depth and rate of respiration followed by respiratory decreases (Cheyne-Stokes

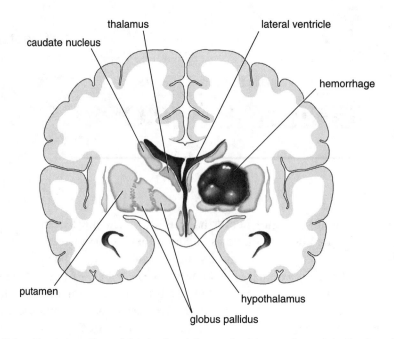

caudate nucleus

thalamus

lateral ventricle

hemorrhage

putamen

hypothalamus

globus pallidus

Figure 6-1. Frontal section of the brain. Intracerebral hemorrhage into the basal ganglia. Note that the extravasated blood forms a mass that displaces midline structures.

respiration) also are more characteristic of hemorrhage than ischemia. With hypertensive hemorrhages, bleeding does not usually occur again into the same area.

Extravasated blood is not removed quickly from brain tissue. Weeks or months may be required. Neurologic deficits thus recover slowly. About 30 to 35 percent of patients die within 1 to 30 days. This is due to the hemorrhage extending into the ventricular system, to the herniation of the temporal lobe which compresses the midbrain, or to both. With smaller hemorrhages, there may be a considerable recovery of function. To some extent this is due to the fact that a small hemorrhage pushes brain tissue aside rather than destroying it.

STROKE SYNDROMES

CT scanning, a highly useful technique for the diagnosis of primary intracerebral hemorrhage, has shown that spontaneous bleeding can occur in almost any part of the brain. However, certain areas of the central nervous system (CNS) are favored sites. About 60 percent of primary intracerebral hemorrhages occur into the putamen and adjacent internal capsule due to rupture of the penetrating branches of the middle cerebral artery (the lenticulostriate arteries, also called the arteries of hemorrhage) (Figure 6-2). The second most common site is hemorrhage into the posterior portions of the thalamus and is due to rupture of the penetrating branches of the posterior cerebral artery. Less common sites are hemorrhage into the central pons and deeper portions of the cerebellum (Figure 6-3). Hemorrhages may also occur into the subcortical white matter. Ocular signs (reactivity of the pupils to light and position of the eyeball) are important in localizing the site of intracerebral hemorrhage.

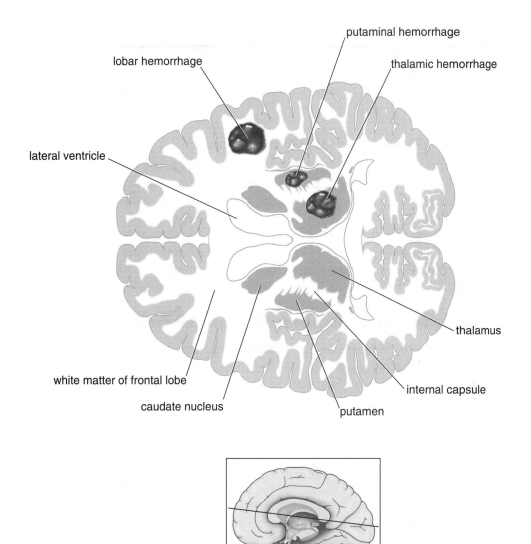

Figure 6-2. Horizontal section through the cerebral hemispheres illustrating hemorrhages into the putamen, thalamus, and lobe of the hemisphere.

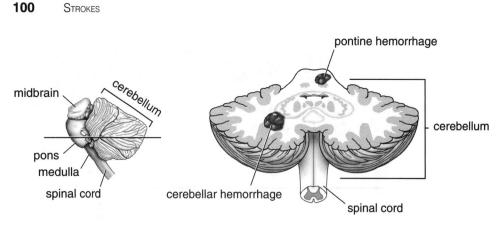

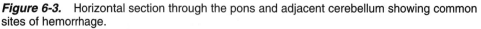

Figure 6-3.   Horizontal section through the pons and adjacent cerebellum showing common sites of hemorrhage.

Basal Ganglia–Internal Capsule Hemorrhage

The basal ganglia include the caudate nucleus, the putamen, and the globus pallidus. The prognosis for survival and recovery relate to the size of the hemorrhage. Large hemorrhages produce signs of upper brain stem compression including coma, compromise of respiratory function, dilated and fixed pupils unresponsive to light, and occasionally decerebrate rigidity. Death occurs in about 75 percent of such patients within a matter of hours or days. Smaller hemorrhages result in proportionately fewer neurologic signs and symptoms. Sometimes considerable recovery may occur over time.

   Typical symptoms of hemorrhage into the basal ganglia include:

- A sudden onset of headache followed shortly (5 to 30 minutes) by a progressive contralateral hemiparesis.
- The face sags on one side, speech becomes slurred or aphasic, and the arm and leg gradually weaken.
- The hemiparesis is often accompanied by a deviation of the eyes away from the side of the hemiparesis.
- The patient usually is confused.
- Continued bleeding causes a worsening of signs and symptoms.
   - Paralysis worsens, bilateral Babinski signs develop, speech becomes impossible, the patient becomes unresponsive to painful stimuli (hemianesthesia), and stupor develops.

Thalamic Hemorrhage

The prognosis for survival and recovery relate to the size of the hemorrhage. Large hemorrhages are usually fatal. Hemorrhages of moderate size produce:

- Contralateral hemiparesis or hemiplegia due to compression of the internal capsule.

- Contralateral loss of sensation, which equals or exceeds in severity the motor weakness.
- Ocular signs are common due to extension of the hemorrhage into the brain stem and include defects in upward gaze, deviation of the eyes down and laterally at rest, inequality of pupillary size and an absence of light reflexes, as well as other signs of ocular dysfunction.

Pontine Hemorrhage

Hemorrhage into the pons generally is fatal. The rare cases that survive usually remain quadriplegic and dependent upon caregivers. Onset of the hemorrhage is usually marked by a sudden headache. The headache is followed within seconds or minutes by a number of signs and symptoms:

- Total paralysis (tetraplegia).
- Decerebrate rigidity.
- Pin-point pupils (1 mm) with preserved light reflexes.
- Impaired or absent lateral eye movements (bilateral conjugate gaze paralysis).
- Ocular bobbing (a fast jerk of the eyes in a downward direction followed by a slow drift to the midposition).
- Impaired breathing.

Cerebellar Hemorrhage

Cerebellar hemorrhages are often characterized by the sudden onset of headache in the occipital region on the side of the bleeding. The symptoms usually develop over a period of hours.

- Classic signs of cerebellar involvement may be seen at the outset.
  - □ These include nystagmus and ataxia, but such signs are not present in all cases.
- Vertigo and disequilibrium result in an inability to sit, stand, or walk.
- There is paralysis of conjugate lateral gaze to the side of the lesion or an ipsilateral sixth nerve weakness resulting in diplopia.
- Ipsilateral facial weakness often occurs with a loss of the corneal reflex.
- Dysarthria and dysphagia may occur.
- Some of these signs are due to compression of the pons caused by the hemorrhagic mass.
- Compression of the brain stem also may result in the patient becoming comatose and developing signs of spastic paralysis in the legs (paraparesis) or all four extremities (quadraplegia).

Lobar Hemorrhage

Hemorrhages may occur into various parts of the central white matter of the frontal, temporal, parietal, and occipital lobes. Such hemorrhages may produce few symptoms, or deficits that resemble those following ischemic stroke. These so-called lobar hemorrhages are readily visualized in a CT scan. They are usually associated with a progressively worsening headache, vomiting, and drowsiness.

TREATMENT

The deep location of hemorrhages into the putamen, thalamus, and pons means that surgical removal of the clot is not feasible. As noted, hemorrhage into the pons is usually fatal as is extension of a thalamic or putaminal hemorrhage into the ventricles of the brain. When diagnosed prior to brain stem compression, patients with cerebellar hemorrhage may be treated surgically as a life-saving measure. Patients in deep coma with dilated fixed pupils seldom survive and nothing can be done to help.

Chapter 7

RUPTURED INTRACRANIAL ANEURYSMS

Aruptured intracranial aneurysm is the fourth most common cause of stroke in adults. The source of the bleeding is a ruptured saccular, or berry, aneurysm. Berry aneurysms are small localized balloonings, or dilations, of a vessel wall resulting from a defect in the elasticity of the vessel. The vast majority, 90 to 95 percent, occur in relation to the anterior portion of the circle of Willis located at the base of the brain. The aneurysms occur at points of bifurcation or branching (Figure 7-1). Only some 10 percent occur in relation to the vertebral-basilar system.

The unruptured saccular aneurysm usually causes no focal signs or symptoms. Notable exceptions to this are aneurysms that compress the optic nerves or chiasm, the hypothalamus, the pituitary gland, or the third, fourth, fifth, or sixth cranial nerves. Unruptured saccular aneurysms occur as an incidental finding in 2 percent of routine autopsies.

Rupture can occur at any age but is most common between the ages of 40 and 65 years. In most cases there are no warning symptoms of an impending rupture. Most ruptures occur during the waking hours, often precipitated by straining, exercise, or sexual activity.

Except as noted, initial symptoms are related to rupture of the aneurysm when blood is forced into the subarachnoid space in which the circle of Willis is located. The usual symptoms include:

- Sudden severe headache, vomiting, neck pain and stiffness, and loss of consciousness.
- Neck pain and stiffness at the outset imply a large hemorrhage.
- Blood from the ruptured aneurysm may do one or any combination of the following:
  - It may stay confined to the subarachnoid space (Figure 3-1B).
  - In 30–40 percent of cases, blood extends into the substance of the brain (Figure 7-2B).
  - It may extend into a brain ventricle.

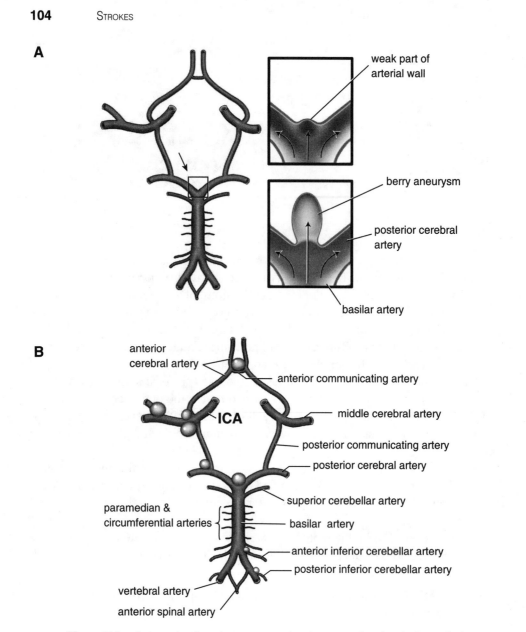

A

weak part of
arterial wall

berry aneurysm

posterior cerebral
artery

basilar artery

B

anterior
cerebral artery

anterior communicating artery

middle cerebral artery

ICA

posterior communicating artery

posterior cerebral artery

superior cerebellar artery

paramedian &
circumferential arteries

basilar artery

anterior inferior cerebellar artery

posterior inferior cerebellar artery

vertebral artery

anterior spinal artery

Figure 7-1. A, saccular (berry) aneurysms develop at weak points in the wall of an artery. Over time, especially in people with high blood pressure, the weak part of the vessel wall expands. B, saccular aneurysms occur at common sites. The size of the aneurysm approximates the frequency at that site. About 90 percent of aneurysms occur on the anterior half of the circle of Willis. Abbreviation: ICA, internal carotid artery.

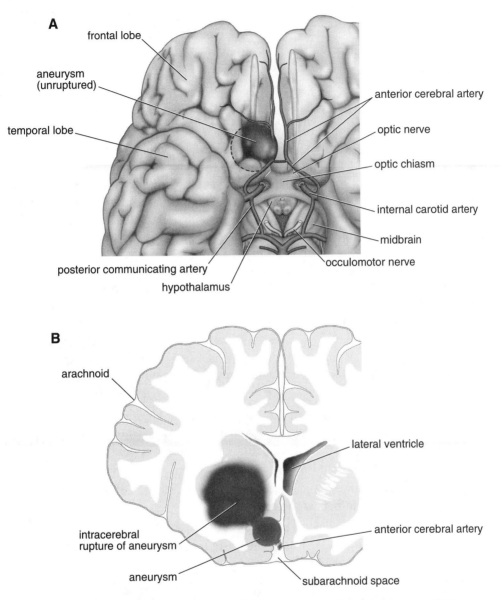

Figure 7-2. A, ventral view of the brain showing an unruptured aneurysm of the anterior cerebral artery. B, frontal section of the brain showing that the aneurysm has ruptured intracerebrally.

- Large hemorrhages can produce coma immediately because the bleeding extends into the brain or ruptures into the ventricular system.
- When the hemorrhage is massive, death may occur in a matter of minutes, hours, or in a day or two.
  - □ The patient remains in a deep coma, which is accompanied by irregular respiration and finally respiratory and circulatory collapse.

Less severe bleeding may or may not produce focal signs with lateralizing value. When bleeding is less severe, consciousness is regained within a matter of minutes or hours, but the patient may remain confused and drowsy for days with a severe headache. When the bleeding stays confined to the subarachnoid space, there may be few lateralizing signs, for example, there is no hemiparesis, hemiplegia, homonymous hemianopsia, or aphasia. There are then no clinical signs to point to the actual site of rupture.

The occurrence of focal neurologic signs of cerebral involvement is due to infarction in the territory of the brain supplied by the artery in which the ruptured aneurysm is located. The vessel beyond the point of rupture can be deprived of blood with a resultant infarction within its territory. Alternatively, the presence of subarachnoid blood surrounding an artery may cause an arterial spasm (vasospasm). The resultant vasoconstriction may be severe enough to produce ischemia and infarction within the territory supplied by the vessel. Such focal deficits may resolve in a matter of days indicating that hemorrhage into brain tissue was not responsible for them.

Some patients have focal neurologic signs that do point to the location of the aneurysm (Figure 7-1):

- Ptosis, diplopia, dilation of the pupil, and deviation of one eye laterally (divergent strasbismus) are caused by involvement of the third cranial nerve and indicate an aneurysm at the junction of the posterior communicating artery and the internal carotid artery.
- Monocular blindness suggests an aneurysm at the origin of the ophthalmic artery from the internal carotid artery.
- Transient paresis of one or both legs at the onset of the bleeding indicates an anterior communicating artery aneurysm that has interfered with blood supply in the territories of the ACAs.
- Hemiparesis or an aphasia indicates an aneurysm at the bifurcation of the left middle cerebral artery into superior and inferior divisions.
- After the first day, the development of new focal neurological deficits usually is attributable to a new episode of bleeding.

CLINICAL COURSE AND PROGNOSIS

Between 15 to 22 percent of patients die in relation to the first episode of bleeding. Many of these patients never reach a hospital. Others arrive at a treatment center in a stuperous or comatose state. Of those patients who survive the initial episode of bleeding, the most prominent feature of subarachnoid hemorrhage is the tendency for rebleeding to occur. Rebleeding has been estimated to occur in 30 to 50 percent of patients during the first year following the initial hemorrhage. The first two weeks after hemorrhage onset carry the greatest risk of rebleeding. The mortality associated with rebleeding is high and has been estimated to range from 42 to 80 percent. The prognosis is worst in those patients who are unconscious or poorly responsive.

TREATMENT

The site of the ruptured aneurysm needs to be localized as soon as possible, first with CT scanning and then angiography. When the CT scan is positive, there is no need to perform a cerebrospinal fluid (CSF) analysis. However, when the CT scan is negative, CSF should be examined for the presence of gross blood. Four-vessel cerebral angiography is carried out as soon as possible and within 24 hours of onset.

When an aneurysm is found in a surgically accessible location and the patient is in a suitable clinical condition, definitive treatment consists of surgical clipping or ligating the neck of the leaking aneurysm (Figure 7-3). Surgical procedures carry a definite risk of causing even more brain damage. However, it has been shown that patients whose clinical condition stabilizes to the point where they can be operated upon do better than those who are managed without surgery. The operative mortality is 2 to 3 percent.

In the acute stage of subarachnoid hemorrhage, a variety of treatments may be applied: strict bed rest in a darkened room; administration of benzodiazepine sedatives to maintain rest and quiet; administration of codeine for headache; administration of stool softeners or enemas to prevent straining; maintenance of nearly normal blood pressure with appropriate medication; and fluid administration to maintain normal blood volume.

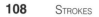

posterior communicating artery

basilar artery

aneurysm clip

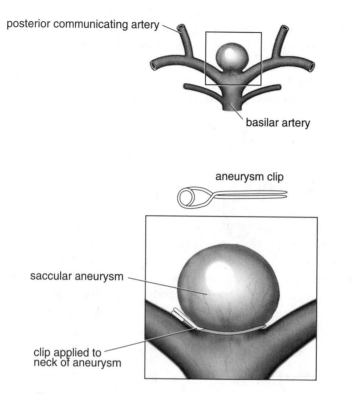

saccular aneurysm

clip applied to
neck of aneurysm

Figure 7-3. Obliteration of an aneurysm by the application of a clip to its neck.

Chapter 8

ARTERIOVENOUS MALFORMATIONS

Arteriovenous malformations (AVMs) consist of a tangle of dilated blood vessels that form an abnormal communication between the arterial and venous systems. AVMs can occur in any part of the brain, brain stem, or spinal cord. They are only one-tenth as common as saccular aneurysms. There are three distinct components of AVMs (Figure 8-1): First, are the arteries that feed into the AVM. Second, is the core, or nidus, which is composed of a snakelike vascular tangle of abnormally thin-walled blood vessels. The core shunts blood directly from the feeding arteries to the third component of the AVM, the draining veins.

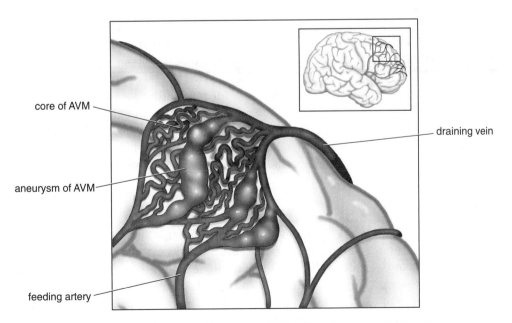

core of AVM

draining vein

aneurysm of AVM

feeding artery

Figure 8-1. Arteriovenous malformation (AVM) with aneurysm. This AVM is illustrated on the surface of the cerebral cortex. However, most large AVMs occur in the central part of a cerebral hemisphere. Components of the AVM are indicated. See text.

The tangled blood vessels of the core may proliferate and enlarge with time. This explains why AVMs most often produce their symptoms in patients over the age of 30 years. AVMs vary in size from a few millimeters in diameter to large masses that may occupy most of the lobe of a cerebral hemisphere. Most large AVMs occur in a cerebral hemisphere at the junction points of the major cerebral arteries.

Many AVMs produce no symptoms for a long time. In the process of their slow growth, large AVMs may produce slowly progressive neurologic deficits because of compression of neighboring structures by the enlarging mass of vessels.

Most AVMs eventually hemorrhage because of the thinness of the walls of blood vessels composing the core of the AVM. While the initial hemorrhage may be fatal, in more than 90 percent of patients the bleeding stops and the patient survives. Prior to rupture, the patient often experiences a chronic, nondescript headache, but in about 10 percent of patients the unilateral headache resembles a classic migraine symptom.

There are three common presenting characteristics of AVMs: hemorrhage, seizure, and headache. As many as half of AVMs leak intermittently, producing various-sized hemorrhages that are partly intracerebral and partly into the subarachnoid space. The intracerebral hemorrhage may cause focal neurological deficits such as a hemiparesis or hemiplegia. While hemorrhage is the most common and dangerous presentation of AVMs, the risk of major neurologic deficits (30 percent) and mortality (15 percent) is lower than with rupture of a saccular aneurysm. In about 30 percent of patients, a focal seizure may be the only manifestation. In another 20 percent of patients, a headache is the only symptom.

A number of diagnostic and imaging studies may be done. Cerebral angiography will demonstrate AVMs larger than 5 mm in diameter and will reveal all three anatomical components of the AVM. CT scans will show AVMs in about 95 percent of patients but CT scanning has become less useful since the advent of magnetic resonance imaging (MRI). MRI reveals AVMs in nearly all cases. MRI is more valuable than cerebral angiography in disclosing the relationship of the AVM to adjacent brain tissue, especially brain tissue that is neurologically indispensable (see following). AVMs that are revealed by MRI or arteriography but cause no symptoms are not treated because the risk of neurologic damage and fatal bleeding is relatively low.

TREATMENT

Surgical removal of the AVM and associated hematoma is the preferred treatment when the lesion is in a surgically accessible area and does not involve areas of the brain that are neurologically indispensable such as the language areas. Surgery can be delayed 2 to 4 weeks allowing the patient to stabilize. Delay is possible because the relative incidence of early rebleeding and delayed neurologic deterioration due to vasospasm is much lower following AVM rupture than following rupture of an aneurysm. Early surgery is necessary only when the hematoma itself warrants surgical evacuation.

Treatment risk can be assessed accurately because the natural history of AVMs is fairly well known. An accurate preoperative assessment of the risks of treatment for a given AVM allows the physician to weigh the risks of surgical intervention against the anticipated clinical course of the lesion. A number of AVM grading schemes have been proposed that use the characteristics of the AVM (size, location, and pattern of venous drainage) to predict the surgical risk. Some AVMs carry a very low surgical risk, others carry a 20 to 22 percent risk of causing neurologic deficits, while still others are inoperable. Surgical efforts to reduce the size of the AVM by ligation or occlusion of the feeding arteries may be made prior to the removal of the AVM.

Radiation (radiosurgery) of the AVM may be done. However, the AVM must be completely obliterated for the treatment to be fully successful since the annual rate of hemorrhage from an AVM does not diminish until it has become completely obliterated. It requires years for radiosurgical treatment to become fully successful during which time the patient is relatively unprotected. Radiosurgery is most successful in the treatment of small AVMs that are deeply located. In such cases, the AVM will be obliterated in 80 to 85 percent of cases after two years. The additional two years of risk for hemorrhage and the 15 to 20 percent rate of failure of total obliteration may make the initial advantages of radiosurgery insufficient to replace conventional surgery.

SELECTED BIBLIOGRAPHY

Adams, R.D., Victor, M., Ropper, A.H., *Principles of Neurology,* 6th edition. New York: McGraw-Hill, 1997.

Barnett, H.J.M., Mohr, J.P., Stein, B.M., Yalsu, F.M. (eds), *Stroke: Pathophysiology, Diagnosis, Management,* 2nd edition. New York: Churchill Livingston, Inc., 1992.

Brodal, A., *Neurological Anatomy in Relation to Clinical Medicine,* 3rd edition. New York: Oxford University Press, 1981.

Brott, T., Thrombolysis for stroke. *Arch. Neurol.,* 53:1305, 1996.

Duvernoy, H.M., *The Human Brainstem and Cerebellum: Surface, Structure, Vascularization and Three-dimensional Sectional Anatomy with MRI.* New York: SpringerWein, 1995.

Duvernoy, H.M., *The Human Brain: Surface, Blood Supply, and Three-dimensional Sectional Anatomy,* 2nd edition. New York: SpringerWein, 1999.

Guthkelch, A.N., and Misulis, K.E. (eds), *The Scientific Foundations of Neurology.* Cambridge: Blackwell Science, Inc., 1996.

Mohr, J.P., and Gautier, J.C. (eds), *Guide to Clinical Neurology.* New York: Churchill Livingston, Inc., 1995.

Parent, A., *Carpenter's Human Neuroanatomy*, 9th edition. Baltimore: Williams & Wilkins, 1996.

Roberts, M., and Hanaway, J., *Atlas of the Human Brain in Section.* Philadelphia: Lea & Febiger, 1971.

Ross, R.W. (ed), *Vascular Diseases of the Central Nervous System,* 2nd edition. New York: Churchill Livingston, Inc., 1983.

Tatu, L., Moulin, T., Bogousslavsky, J., Duvernoy, H., Arterial territories of the human brain: brainstem and cerebellum. *Neurology,* 47: 1125, 1996.

Toole, J.F., *Cerebrovascular Disorders,* 4th edition. New York: Raven Press, 1990.

Vinken, P.J., Bruyn, G.W., Klawans, H.L. (eds), *Handbook of Clinical Neurology, vol. 53, Vascular Diseases.* Amsterdam: Elsevier, 1988.

World Health Organization, *International Classification of Impairments, Disabilities, and Handicaps.* WHO, Geneva, 1980.

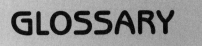

GLOSSARY

A

Abdominal (skin, cutaneous) reflex   Contraction of the muscles of the abdominal wall so that the umbilicus (belly button) is drawn slightly toward the site of the gentle scratch stimulus on the skin.

Abducens   The sixth cranial nerve that supplies the lateral rectus muscle, which moves the eyeball to the side, away from the midline.

Abulia   A state in which the patient manifests a quantitative reduction in spontaneity, initiative, thoughts per unit of time, spoken words, and emotional reaction (apathy). All actions are performed slowly. It is a sign of frontal lobe damage.

Acalculia   Difficulties in calculating.

Accessory nerve   The cranial root of the eleventh cranial nerve supplies motor fibers to the muscles of the larynx. The spinal root supplies motor fibers to the sternocleidomastoid and upper parts of the trapezius muscles.

Acute   A disease of short and well-defined course.

Adiadochokinesis   The inability to perform rapid alternating movements. A characteristic sign of damage to the cerebellum.

Affect   The range, depth, and appropriateness of a person's emotional responses.

Ageusia   Loss of the sense of taste.

Agnosia   Impairment of the ability to recognize stimuli that were formerly recognized, not due to disturbances of perception, intelligence, or language.

Agonist   A muscle whose action is to produce the particular movement in question.

Agraphesthesia   Loss of the ability to identify letters, figures, or numbers drawn on the surface of the skin.

Agraphia   Inability to write due to a cerebral lesion but not due to a motor disability.

Akathisia   A strong subjective feeling of inner restlessness or an irresistible urge to be in constant motion, of which the patient is very aware.

Akinesia   A movement disorder characterized by poverty and slowness of initiation and execution of voluntary movements, and difficulty in changing one motor pattern to another in the absence of paralysis.

Akinesthesia   Loss of the ability to detect the direction of movement of a body part.

Akinetic mutism   A state in which the patient appears to be awake but is motionless (akinetic) and mute.

Alalia   Loss of the power of speech due to paralysis of the vocal apparatus.

Alertness   A state in which the subject is awake and responsive to all environmental stimuli.

Alexia   Loss of the ability to comprehend the meaning of written language symbols.

Alexia without agraphia   An inability to read letters, words, or musical notation and often to name colors. Understanding spoken language, repetition of what is heard, and writing spontaneously and to dictation are preserved.

Alien hand syndrome   Autonomous movements of a limb that are perceived by the patient as being outside of his control.

Allodynia   Pain resulting from a stimulus that does not normally cause pain.

Alogia   Inability to speak.

Alternating hemiplegia   Paresis of cranial nerves on one side of the body and of the limbs and trunk on the other caused by a lesion of the brain stem.

Amaurosis fugax   Temporary blindness in one eye due to occlusion of the ophthalmic artery. More commonly referred to as **transient monocular blindness**.

Amnesia   The loss of memories or an inability to form new ones in a patient who is alert and responsive.

Amnestic   A term for diseases causing a loss of memory.

Amnestic confabulatory syndrome   See **Korsakoff Syndrome**.

Amorphosynthesis   A disorder of the awareness of extrapersonal space and neglect of one side of the body.

Analgesia   Insensitivity to pain, or lack of pain sensation.

Anarthria   Loss of the ability to articulate speech sounds.

Anastomosis   A natural communication between two blood vessels.

Anergy   Lack of strength or vigor.

Anesthesia   Loss of all sensation.

Aneurysm   A local expansion in the diameter of an artery due to a defect in its wall.

Angiography   Techniques for visualizing the anatomy and pathology of the arterial system by means of the injection of radio-opaque dyes with x-ray imaging or magnetic resonance imaging.

Angioma   A vascular malformation including **arteriovenous malformations** and others.

Anhedonia   Loss of the power of enjoyment and inability to experience pleasure.

Anhydrosis   Absence of sweating.

Anisocoria   Inequality in the diameter of the two pupils.

Anomia   The inability to recall and produce names. Present in all forms of aphasia.

Anomic aphasia   A defect in naming, the most common form of aphasia.

Anosmia   Loss of the sense of smell.

Anosoagnosia   Unawareness of the presence of disease ranging from a simple lack of concern about an admitted defect to denial of ownership of a paralyzed limb. Seen most often with lesions of the right parietal lobe, in which case the patient is unaware about deficits on the left side of the body.

Anterograde amnesia   Loss of the ability to learn new material.

Anticoagulant   An agent to prevent coagulation of the blood.

Antiplatelet drugs   Platelets are cell fragments present in blood and are normally involved in blood clotting following vascular injury. They also participate in reactions that lead to atherosclerosis and thrombosis. Antagonists of platelet function (antiplatelet drugs) inhibit the action of platelets. They are used following transient ischemic attacks and minor strokes to prevent (prophylaxis) further TIAs and strokes. Aspirin and ticlopidine are antiplatelet drugs.

Anton Syndrome   Anosognosia for blindness or denial of blindness following bilateral occipital lobe damage.

Apathy   Lack of emotion and indifference with reduced activity. A sign of frontal and temporal lobe damage.

Aphasia   A disturbance in the uses of language due to cerebral injury and not due to sensory or motor disturbances or to generalized mental deterioration. See **Broca's aphasia, Wernicke's aphasia**.

Aphemia   A term originally used by neurologist Paul Broca to describe loss of the ability to speak. The term *Broca's aphasia* is now preferred.

Aphonia   Loss of the ability to produce vocal sounds or to phonate.

Apnea   Cessation of breathing.

Apoplexy   An obsolete term for stroke.

Apraxia   An inability to carry out on request or by imitation a complex voluntary movement not due to paralysis, paresis, ataxia, sensory changes, or deficiencies of understanding.

Aprosody (Aprosodia)   Loss of **prosody** in speech. The term *prosody* describes the melodious aspect of speech with an emphasis on stress (inflection), pitch (tone), timbre, and rhythm.

Arachnoid   The thin middle layer of the three meninges surrounding the central nervous system.

Arteriography   See **angiography**.

Arteriole   A small terminal artery continuous with a capillary network.

Artery   A blood vessel that carries blood away from the heart and toward a peripheral capillary.

Arteriovenous malformation   An uncommon congenital vascular malformation in which there is direct artery-to-vein communication without an intervening capillary bed. The malformation evolves during life and may hemorrhage.

Arteritis   Inflammatory disease of an artery or arteries.

Asimultagnosia   Inability to perceive the entire visual field at one time, or an inability to appreciate the simultaneous occurrence of tactile or auditory stimuli on each side of the body.

Asomatognosia   Loss of the concept of parts or even one half of the body due to a disorder of the body image or body scheme. Asomatognosias are caused by lesion to the posterior parietal lobes.

Astereognosis   Loss of the ability to identify objects (such as a car key) by manipulation without the use of vision.

Asthenia Generalized weakness and unwillingness to attempt muscular activity.

Asynergy (Asynergia) Lack of cooperation or working together of agonist and antagonist muscles due to disease of the cerebellum.

Ataxia Incoordination or awkwardness in the performance of a motor task. May be due to motor system (cerebellar) or sensory system lesions.

Ataxic gait A wide-based, lurching gait in which steps are taken irregularly and are of unequal length.

Ataxic tremor See **cerebellar tremor**.

Atherothrombotic infarction Infarction of the brain due to occlusion of a supplying artery by a combination of atherosclerosis and clot formation at the site of the atherosclerotic plaque.

Athetosis Involuntary movements that are more or less continuous, slow, writhing movements of any combination of abduction and adduction, flexion and extension, and pronation and supination in varying degree. The movements blend with one another to give the appearance of a continuous, mobile spasm. In general, these purposeless movements are most pronounced in the fingers and hands, face, and tongue, but all muscles may be involved.

Atonia Muscle tone is the slight resistance that a normal relaxed muscle offers to passive movement. In atonia, muscle tone is reduced or absent.

Attention The capacity to concentrate upon one of a number of competing stimuli or to maintain a readiness to respond to a specific stimulus without being distracted by extraneous stimuli.

Audiometry Techniques for the quantitative measurement of hearing acuity.

Auditory agnosia A disorder in the recognition of sounds (verbal or nonverbal) in a patient with normal hearing, alertness, and intelligence.

Autonomic nervous system Nuclei, tracts, ganglia, and nerves of the central and peripheral nervous systems involved in the unconscious regulation of visceral functions.

Autotopagnosia Difficulty in localizing and naming one's own body parts.

Axon The part of a nerve cell involved in conducting action potentials.

B

Babinski sign Consists of upward (dorsiflexion) of the big toe and lateral fanning of the other toes in response to uncomfortable stimulation of the sole of the foot. A sign indicative of damage to the pyramidal tract.

Balance The ability to maintain an upright posture during sitting, standing, and walking by detecting and correcting displacements from the line of gravity beyond the base of support.

Balint Syndrome Consists of an inability to direct the eyes to a certain point in the visual field despite the retention of intact eye movements, a disorder of grasping or touching an object under visual guidance (optic ataxia), and fluctuating visual inattention for any stimulus not exciting the macula of the retina.

Ballism A term used to describe the involuntary abrupt contraction of the axial and proximal muscles of the extremities. The contractions are sufficiently violent to result in a flailing about of the extremities. Ballism usually is confined to one side of the body (**hemiballismus, hemiballism**) and is due to a lesion of the subthalamic nucleus.

Baresthesia The sense of weight or pressure.

Barognosis The ability to discriminate between different weights.

Basal ganglia Deep nuclei of the cerebrum concerned with the elaboration of motor activity and certain aspects of cognition and emotion. They include the caudate, putamen, globus pallidus, substantia nigra, subthalamic nucleus, and amygdala.

Benedikt Syndrome Oculomotor palsy with contralateral cerebellar ataxia, tremor, and corticospinal tract signs due to a lesion of the tegmentum of the midbrain.

Biceps reflex Contraction of the biceps muscle in response to a tap over its tendon. The reflex is elicited by placing the examiner's index finger over the biceps tendon and tapping the finger.

Bilateral On both sides.

Blindsight The capacity to look toward unseen targets presented within an area of a visual field defect (blindness, or scotoma) in a patient with damage to the visual cortex.

Blink reflex Closure of the eyes with tactile stimulation of the upper part of the face or with sudden visual stimulation.

Block design test A task in which the subject is required to reproduce a patterned block design in order to match the pattern presented on a card. A subtest of the Wechsler Adult Intelligence Scale.

Blood-brain barrier Mechanisms possessed by the cells of blood vessels in the brain and spinal cord that oppose the passage into the internal environment of the brain (the extracellular fluid) of most ions and large molecules suspended in the blood.

Body scheme A term used to describe a person's conception of the portion of space occupied by his body, the relationship of the parts of the body to one another, and the right and left sides of the body.

Bradykinesia Abnormal slowness in the performance of motor tasks.

Brain That part of the central nervous system controlling our internal environment and all willful and involuntary interactions with the external world.

Brain death The diagnosis of brain death depends on (1) the absence of cerebral functions (absence of all spontaneous movement and motor and vocal responses to all sensory stimuli), (2) absence of brain stem function, including respiration, and (3) irreversibility of the condition. Brain death is confirmed by electroencephalography.

Brain herniation The protrusion of brain tissue through the tissues normally containing it. Brain herniation becomes possible because the cranial cavity is subdivided into several compartments by relatively rigid sheets of dura mater. The pressure from a mass lesion within one compartment is not evenly distributed so brain tissue shifts from the compartment where the pressure is higher to another compartment where it is lower.

Brain stem   That part of the central nervous system consisting of the medulla, pons, and midbrain.

Broca's aphasia   Also called **motor** or **expressive aphasia**. It is characterized by a reduced verbal output (hypofluent), difficulty initiating speech, slow and effortful articulation, loss of prosody, use of simple grammatical forms in both speech and writing, and normal comprehension of written and spoken language. The causative lesion involves the posterior part of the inferior frontal gyrus in the dominant (usually left) cerebral hemisphere.

Brodmann's areas   Numbered areas of the cerebral cortex distinguished by the occurrence and arrangement of cells in the different layers of the cerebral cortex.

Bruit   An abnormal sound generated as a result of the turbulent flow of blood through an artery that has been narrowed by disease. Bruit is heard with a stethoscope.

Buccofacial apraxia   An inability to perform learned, skilled movements with the facial and bulbar muscles.

Bulbar   Relating to the medulla oblongata of the brain stem.

Bulbar palsy   Weakness of the face and tongue, dysphagia, dysarthria, and dysphonia due to pathology of the lower brain stem (lower pons and medulla) or to the nerves derived from it.

C

Callosal apraxia   Apraxia of the left hand caused by a lesion of fibers of the corpus callosum.

Cardiogenic embolism   Emboli arising from the heart and traveling into the cerebral circulation.

Carotid border syndrome   A syndrome characterized by focal numbness and weakness of the hand caused by partial occlusion of the internal carotid artery.

Carotid sinus   An approximately 1 cm long dilation of the internal carotid artery, containing baroreceptors which send information on blood pressure to the medulla via the ninth cranial nerve.

Central pain   Severe pain of unknown mechanism arising from lesions within the central nervous system.

Central photophobia   A complaint of excessive brightness in a patient with a homonymous hemianopsia as a result of a visual cortex (occipital lobe) lesion.

Central midbrain syndrome   A syndrome resulting from occlusion of the interpeduncular branches of the posterior cerebral artery. The syndrome is characterized oculomotor palsy with contralateral hemiplegia, paralysis of vertical gaze, stupor or coma, and an ataxic tremor.

Cerebellar ataxia   A term that covers all of the movement deficits resulting from cerebellar disease or lesions of the pathways connecting the cerebellum to other parts of the brain. The term refers in particular to incoordination or awkwardness in the performance of a movement.

Cerebellar gait   The main characteristics of this gait are a wide separation of the legs (base-wide), unsteady and irregular steps, and lateral veering.

Cerebellar signs   These include postural hypotonia, pendular knee jerk, asthenia and fatigability, ataxia, decomposition of movement, dysmetria, dysdiadochokinesis, cerebellar tremor, dysarthria, and nystagmus.

Cerebellar tremor   This is called intention tremor even though it is understood that no tremor is intentional. Cerebellar tremors occur with goal-directed voluntary movement and increase in amplitude as the limb approaches the target.

Cerebral apoplexy   Intracerebral hemorrhage.

Cerebral cortex   The outer surface of the brain consisting primarily of glial cells and the cell bodies of neurons. Most of the cerebral cortex is composed of six layers of cells, but the cortex in certain areas of the brain has only three or four layers.

Cerebral dominance   The specialization of one hemisphere for the performance of a specific function. The left hemisphere is dominant for speech in almost all people who are right-handed (over 90 percent) and in most people who are left-handed (about 60 percent). The right hemisphere is dominant for spatial skills and many aspects of emotion.

Cerebral edema   An increase in the volume of the brain due to an increase in the brain's water content. Brain cells (neurons and glia) may themselves swell (cytotoxic edema), as with hypoxia, or the amount of fluid outside of brain cells may increase (vasogenic edema) as with tumors or infarcts.

Cerebral embolism   Occlusion of a cerebral blood vessel by a clot of blood or other material such as cholesterol.

Cerebral hemorrhage   Bleeding into the substance of the brain.

Cerebral infarction   Irreversible damage to brain cells within a region of the brain as a result of ischemia.

Cerebral ischemia   Diminished blood supply to the brain due to mechanical obstruction.

Cerebral perfusion pressure   The difference between the mean arterial pressure and the intracranial pressure.

Cerebral thrombosis   The occlusion of an artery by a blood clot that causes ischemia and possible infarction in the brain tissue supplied by the vessel.

Cerebrospinal fluid (CSF)   A clear, colorless fluid that fills the cavities inside the brain (ventricles) and surrounds the brain and spinal cord externally. It is continuously secreted by the choroid plexus and protects and supports the brain and spinal cord.

Cerebrovascular accident (CVA)   See **stroke**.

Cheyne-Stokes respiration   A pattern of respiration with a gradual increase in depth and rate to a maximum and then declining in force and length until breathing stops (apnea). The cycles may last from 30 seconds to 2 minutes, with the apnea lasting from 5 to 30 seconds.

Chiasm   The decussation of fibers of the optic nerves.

Chorea   Brief, involuntary, irregular, nonrepetitive movements flowing randomly from one body part to another.

Chronic   A disease of slow progress and long duration.

Circadian rhythm   Relating to biologic rhythms with a cycle of about one day.

Circle of Willis   A connecting circle, or ring, of arteries at the base of the brain. In an anterior to posterior direction, the circle of Willis is formed by the anterior communicating artery, the two anterior cerebral arteries, the two internal carotid arteries, the two posterior communicating arteries, and the two posterior cerebral arteries.

Circumlocution   The use of many words to communicate an idea that could be expressed by a few words or only one.

Clasp-knife reaction   Often observed in spasticity, the sudden melting away of increased resistance to passive stretch of a muscle like a pocket-knife opening (the give-way phase to extension of the arm) or closing (the give-way phase to flexing the leg).

Clinical   Refers to the symptoms and course of a disease, as distinguished from the laboratory findings.

Clonic   Characterized by alternate contraction and relaxation of muscle.

Clonus   Rhythmical reflex contractions and relaxations of a muscle in response to a sudden maintained stretching force.

Cognition   A generic, imprecise term covering a diverse collection of mental abilities including conceiving, perceiving, memory, use of language, judgment, problem solving, abstraction ability, reasoning, and imagining.

Collateral   A side branch of a blood vessel or axon of a nerve cell.

Collateral circulation   The alternate pathways for blood supply to the brain.

Coma   A state of deep unconsciousness from which the patient cannot be roused.

Comatose   In a state of coma.

Commissure   Nerve fibers that join the two cerebral hemispheres together, such as the corpus callosum.

Communicating hydrocephalus   A poor term designating a form of hydrocephalus in which cerebrospinal fluid formed in the brain ventricles drains into the subarachnoid space but is not reabsorbed into the venous system. Also called *external hydrocephalus*.

Completed stroke   A stroke syndrome in which there is no further progression of signs and symptoms.

Complete basilar syndrome   Results from bilateral occlusion of both the paramedian and circumferential branches of the basilar artery.

Compound movements   Those movements that involve the action of muscles across two or more joints, such as touching the nose with the index finger.

Computerized tomography (CT)   A series of very narrow beams of x-rays are projected through the head onto detection crystals located on the opposite side of the head. The differing densities of bone, CSF, blood, and gray and white matter affect the x-ray beams differently. Computer analysis results in a two-dimensional reconstruction of the brain structures irradiated.

Concentration   The capacity to maintain focused attention upon one task or one object over time.

Concussion   The most common neurological syndrome resulting from trauma to the head and consisting of a transient impairment of consciousness and alteration of higher cerebral function. The mechanism is unknown.

Conduction aphasia   A form of aphasia in which comprehension is preserved, spontaneous speech and writing are fluent and copious with paraphasic errors, and there is a serious impairment in the ability to repeat spoken speech. As in all forms of aphasia, there are word-finding and naming impairments.

Confabulation   The fabrication of information by a patient who believes the statements to be true.

Confabulatory Syndrome   See **Korsakoff Syndrome**.

Confusional state   A mental state in which there is an impaired ability to think with customary clarity and speed. Notable characteristics include lack of coherence in the stream of thought, difficulty with problem solving, impaired judgment, lack of insight, and disorientation.

Congenital   A condition existing at birth that may be either hereditary or due to an influence occurring during gestation up to the time of birth.

Conjugate   The symmetrical and synchronous movement of the two eyes.

Consciousness   That mental state everyone knows and understands until they attempt to define it. To the physician, it is defined as the patient's awareness of self and environment.

Consensus reflex   The occurrence of pupillary contraction in one eye when a light is shown in the opposite eye.

Constructional apraxia   A deficit in the ability to construct the copy of a visually presented model by means of assembling objects or drawing. Despite the name, this is not really an apraxia.

Continence   The ability to maintain voluntary closure of the urinary and anal sphincter.

Contracture   A term applied to all states of fixed muscle shortening.

Contralateral   A symptom or sign occurring on the side of the body opposite the responsible lesion.

Contrecoup injury   A contusion or laceration of the brain on the side opposite to the one that received the blow.

Contusion   A local area of swelling and capillary hemorrhage of the central nervous system resembling a bruise.

Convergence   A turning inward of both eyes when focusing on an object brought near to the face.

Convulsion   A forceful involuntary contraction or spasm of voluntary muscle due to a seizure.

Corneal reflex   The corneal reflex is tested by having the patient look to one side while the cornea is lightly touched with cotton wool. The normal response to this stimulus is a prompt closure of both eyelids. The afferent portion of the reflex is mediated by a branch of the trigeminal (Vth) nerve, while the efferent portion of the reflex is mediated by the facial (VIIth) nerve.

Corpus callosum   The largest set of nerve fibers (8 cm long) interconnecting the two cerebral hemispheres.

Cortical blindness   Loss of vision due to bilateral lesions of the occipital lobes. The visual loss is usually not complete.

Cortical dementia   Memory loss, impaired manipulation of acquired knowledge, concept formation, and set shifting in the presence of prominent aphasia, apraxia, and agnosia.

Cortical sensory syndrome   A defect of sensory discrimination. The patient exhibits an impairment or loss of the following: the ability to distinguish objects by their size, shape, and texture (astereognosis); to recognize figures written on the skin (agraphesthesia); to distinguish between single and double contacts (two-point discrimination); the sense of position and passive movement; and the ability to localize tactile, thermal, or noxious stimuli applied to the body surface. The perception of touch, pressure, pain, thermal, and vibratory stimuli is relatively intact. The lesion is in the postcentral gyrus of the contralateral parietal lobe.

Coumadin   See **Warfarin.**

Cranial nerves   Those nerves exiting the skull and originating from the brain stem or brain.

Cremasteric reflex   Elevation of one testicle in response to scratching the inside of the thigh on the same side.

CT scan   See **computerized tomography**.

Cutaneous reflexes   Reflex motor activity in response to stimulation of the skin or mucous membranes.

Cyanosis   A bluish or purplish color of the skin or mucous membranes due to the presence of deoxygenated blood in vessels near the body surface.

Cyanotic   Pertaining to or marked by cyanosis.

Cytotoxic cerebral edema   Swelling of neuronal and glial cells of the brain due to the accumulation of intracellular water.

D

Decerebrate rigidity   An extensor posture of the neck, trunk, and limbs, and clinching of the jaws with internal rotation of the arms and plantar flexion of the feet. The condition results from functional transection of the brain stem such as occurs with temporal lobe herniation and compression of the midbrain.

Declarative memory   The ability to acquire new information about facts or events and requiring the conscious recollection of a particular instance or experience that could only have occurred at a unique time or place.

Decomposition of movement   The jerky performance of voluntary compound movements in which the component parts of the movement are performed separately, joint by joint. A sign of damage to the lateral cerebellum.

Decorticate rigidity   A state of abnormal flexion of the arms and extension of the legs. The condition is caused by lesions of the cerebral white matter, internal capsules, or thalamus.

Deglutition   Swallowing.

Deja vu   The feeling of increased familiarity or of having experienced something previously.

Dejerine-Roussy Syndrome   See **thalamic syndrome**.

Delirium   A state of confusion and clouded consciousness characterized by difficulty in sustaining attention, disordered thinking, perceptual disorders (hallucinations, illusions), alterations in the sleep-wakefulness cycle, impairment of memory, and motor disturbances (restlessness).

Delusion   An incorrect belief maintained in spite of strong evidence to the contrary.

Dementia   An acquired, persistent symptom complex embracing intellectual, behavioral, and personality deterioration that is severe enough to compromise occupational or social performance. Memory impairment is a cardinal feature.

Demyelination   A loss of the myelin sheath surrounding axons of the central and/or peripheral nervous systems. It may result in a complete or partial block of conduction of action potentials along the axon.

Denervation   The cutting off of the nerve supply to a structure thereby causing changes in the function of the structure.

Depression   A reduction in the level of functioning. A clinically observable feeling of dejection and sadness caused by a life experience or as a result of a brain pathology.

Dermatome   The localized area of the skin supplied by the branches of a single spinal nerve.

Diencephalon   A division of the brain customarily divided into the epithalamus, thalamus, and hypothalamus.

Diffuse   As applied to disorders of the nervous system, a pathological process causing the abnormal function of neurons throughout widespread areas of the nervous system resulting in signs and symptoms without localizing value.

Digital subtraction angiography   A refinement of angiographic technique in which a digital computer "subtracts" an image before injection of a contrast medium from the image taken after injection of the contrast medium. The resulting picture is not as good as that obtained with conventional angiography but the procedure is more economical and safer because it permits a great reduction in the amount of dye injected into the patient.

Dilation (Dilatation)   An abnormal widening of an artery.

Diplopia   Double vision. A single stimulus is perceived as two objects because of a lack of parallelism of the ocular axes.

Disconnection syndromes   Syndromes that result from the interruption of pathways that connect different functional areas of the cerebral cortex, either within the same hemisphere or in different hemispheres. These include alexia without agraphia, ideomotor apraxia, transcortical aphasia, and conduction aphasia.

Disorientation   Loss of the sense of familiarity with one's surroundings or an impairment in the ability to localize oneself within a place.

Dissecting aneurysm   Splitting of the wall of an artery due to disease allowing blood to pass for a varying distance between layers of the arterial wall.

Dissociated anesthesia   Loss or impairment of some forms of sensation with retention of other forms of sensation in the same body part.

Distal   The term for those body parts progressively more distant from the midline.

Dominance   The situation in which a given cerebral hemisphere is primarily responsible for a particular function.

Dressing apraxia   Impairment in the ability to match the form of a garment to the form of one's body. Despite the name, the condition is not a true apraxia.

Drug holiday   The withdrawal of a drug for a temporary period used in some patients experiencing adverse side effects from long-term drug treatment.

Dysarthria   An inability to produce normal motor speech patterns due to a lesion in the motor system, nerves, or speech muscles themselves.

Dysdiadochokinesis   Impairment in the normal rhythm, speed, and force of alternating movements such as pronation and supination of the hand. It is an important sign of a cerebellar lesion on the same side as the deficit.

Dysesthesia   Abnormal sensations, such as tingling or prickling feelings, or burning pain occurring either spontaneously or in response to stimuli that are not normally painful.

Dysgeusia   Impairment or distortion of the sense of taste.

Dyskinesia   Abnormal involuntary movements such as tremors, chorea, ballism, and others.

Dyslexia   An inability to read, spell, and write words, despite normal vision and visual recognition.

Dysmetria   The condition in which a limb undershoots or overshoots its intended target as a result of a cerebellar lesion.

Dysnomia.   Difficulty in naming objects.

Dysphagia   Difficulty swallowing.

Dysphasia   See **aphasia**.

Dysprosody   See **aprosody**.

Dystonia   Sustained and patterned contractions of muscles leading to abnormal and twisted postures that may be repeated or fixed and painful.

Dystonic   Pertaining to dystonia.

Dysthymia   A chronic and mild form of depression lasting at least two years.

E

Edema See **cerebral edema**.

EEG Abbreviation for **electroencephalogram**.

Electrocorticogram The record of electroencephalographic activity recorded by means of electrodes applied to the scalp or inserted into the brain.

Electrode Either of the conductors by which an electric current enters or leaves the body. The device used to deliver an electrical current (stimulating electrode) or to record an electrical potential (recording electrode).

Electroencephalogram A record of electrical activity of the brain recorded by means of electrodes applied to the scalp or inserted into the brain.

Electroencephalography The procedure of recording the electrical activity of the brain through electrodes applied to the scalp or inserted into the brain. The analysis of records so obtained.

Electromyogram A record of the electrical activity of muscle recorded by electrodes applied to the skin or inserted into a muscle.

Electromyography The procedure of recording the electrical activity of muscle during rest and movement through electrodes applied to the skin or inserted into a muscle. The analysis of records so obtained.

Electroneuronography The recording and study of action potentials in peripheral nerves elicited in response to electrical or physiological stimuli.

Eloquent cortex The areas of the cerebral cortex devoted to the faculty of speech.

Embolic infarction The area of dead (necrotic) brain cells due to insufficiency of blood supply caused by an embolus.

Embolism Obstruction or occlusion of an artery by an embolus.

Embolus A plug occluding a vessel that has been carried to the site of obstruction in the circulation. The plug may be a detached fragment of a thrombus, cholesterol, or rarely, fat or air.

Emotional lability Unstable emotions that change abruptly without a sufficient stimulus.

Emotional facial palsy A rare condition in which there is a loss of emotional movements (such as laughing) in the lower half of the face, but there is no loss of voluntary movements.

Encephalitis Diffuse inflammation of the substance of the brain.

Encephalon Used as a synonym for *the brain.*

Encephalomalacia A softening of brain tissue, usually due to necrosis of vascular origin.

Encephalopathy Disease of the brain.

Endarterectomy A surgical procedure in which occluding material, such as atherosclerotic deposits, are removed from an artery so as to leave a smooth lining. The procedure increases blood flow and reduces turbulence and future platelet deposition.

End-artery   An artery that is the sole supply to a given area of the brain.

Endocarditis   Inflammation of the endocardium, the innermost layer of the heart. The resulting clots and vegetations often give rise to emboli.

Enteric nervous system   The component of the autonomic nervous system that innervates the gastrointestinal tract, the pancreas, and the gall bladder.

Environmental schema   The representation in the brain of the space around one's body.

Epidemiology   The study of the factors that determine the frequency and distribution of disease in a human or animal population.

Ependyma   The epithelial cells lining the ventricles of the brain and the central canal of the spinal cord.

Epidural hemorrhage   Bleeding outside the dura mater that strips the dura mater from the inner surface of the skull.

Epilepsy   The repeated occurrence of sudden, excessive, and synchronous discharges in large groups of neurons resulting in almost instantaneous disruption of consciousness, disturbance of sensation, convulsive movements, impaired mental function, or some combination of these behavioral signs. A disease of the brain.

Epileptiform   Resembling epilepsy.

Epileptogenic   Capable of causing epileptic seizures.

Evoked potential   An electrical waveform recorded by electrodes in response to an electrical or physiological stimulus applied to the central or peripheral nervous system.

Evolving stroke   The portion of a stroke syndrome in which there is a progression of deficits with time.

Explicit memory   See **declarative memory**.

Expressive aphasia   See **Broca's aphasia**.

Exteroception   Denoting information originating from sensory receptors distributed in the skin and subcutaneous tissues. Examples are touch, pressure, superficial pain, and temperature.

Extradural hemorrhage   See **epidural hemorrhage**.

Extramedullary   Outside the spinal cord.

Extrapyramidal system   The portions of the brain and their pathways that contribute to the control of movement apart from the pyramidal system. It consists of two parts: the basal ganglia and the cerebellum. The distinction between pyramidal and extrapyramidal systems is an anatomical distinction and is without functional significance.

F

Facial palsy   Weakness of the muscles of the face including the periorbital muscles.

Falx cerebri   A sheet of dura mater that separates and supports the two cerebral hemispheres.

Facies   Facial expression.

False localizing sign   A neurological sign that incorrectly suggests the location of a lesion at a particular site in the brain. Tumors often produce such signs.

Fasciculations   Spontaneous contractions of all the myofibrils (muscle cells) making up a motor unit. The twitches can be seen and felt by the subject or an examiner.

Fatigability   The condition following a period of mental or muscular activity in which there is a reduced efficiency of accomplishment or a reduced output of power.

Fatigue   The majority of patients recovering from a stroke complain of being weak and tired.

Feeling tone   See **affect**.

Field of vision (visual field)   The area of space simultaneously visible to one eye without movement.

Figure writing (graphesthesia)   The recognition of letters, numbers, or geometric forms written on the surface of the skin.

Fissure of Rolando   The central fissure of a cerebral hemisphere separating the frontal lobe from the parietal lobe.

Fissure of Sylvius   The lateral fissure of a hemisphere marking the superior extent of the temporal lobe.

Fixation point   The object of vision when both eyes are simultaneously directed to the same target.

Flaccid   Relaxed, flabby, without muscle tone.

Flexion reflex   Dorsiflexion of the big toe with flexion at the ankle, knee, and hip in response to painful stimulation of the foot or leg. It is not elicited in the neurologic exam, but the Babinski reflex is a fragment of this full flexor response and is tested in the neurologic exam.

Fluent aphasia   The type of aphasia characterized by plentiful and often meaningless speech. See **Wernicke's aphasia**.

Focal   As applied to disorders of the nervous system, a pathological process occurring in a single, geographic area of the brain that produces signs and symptoms referable to the function of that area.

Foramen magnum   The large aperture at the base of the skull through which the cranial cavity communicates with the vertebral canal. It houses the uppermost portion of the cervical spinal cord.

Forced laughing and crying   Uncontrollable spasms of hilarious laugher or uncontrollable crying without a sufficient stimulus.

Frontal cortex   Cortex of the frontal lobe, which makes up the anterior one-third of each hemisphere.

G

Gadolinium   A paramagnetic agent that alters the magnetic environment of water and thereby influences the appearance of an MRI. The agent leaks into structures of the brain that lack a blood-brain barrier and makes such areas more conspicuous on an MRI.

Gag reflex   Elevation of the soft palate and contraction of the pharyngeal constrictors by touching the posterior wall of the pharynx with a wooden tongue depressor.

Gait   Manner of walking.

Ganglion   A collection of nerve cell bodies in the peripheral nervous system and excluding the inappropriately named basal ganglia of the central nervous system.

Gaze apraxia   Inability to direct the eyes in response to a command or to a stimulus presented in visual space with no paralysis of eye movement. Seen as a component of the **Balint Syndrome**.

Gaze palsy   A deficit in the conjugate deviation of the eyes in any direction.

Generalized seizure   A seizure in which the entire brain is involved in the seizure discharge at its onset. May be a grand mal (tonic-clonic), absence, atonic, or myotonic seizure.

Genu   A bend resembling a flexed knee in part of an anatomical structure.

Gliosis   Following local brain tissue destruction, a process of structural repair in the CNS in which astrocytes proliferate and produce intracellular filaments resulting in a local increase of neuroglial fibers.

Global aphasia   A type of aphasia in which there is a severe impairment of fluency, comprehension, naming, and repetition. It is a combination of the symptoms of **Broca's** and **Wernicke's aphasias** in which the patient is unable to either formulate speech or comprehend language.

Glossopharyngeal nerve   The IXth cranial nerve that supplies first and foremost the tongue and pharynx.

Gnosis   The ability to know and understand the significance of persons and things that are perceived.

Graphesthesia   The ability to recognize figures and letters written on the skin.

Grasp reflex   Flexion of the fingers over an object placed in the palm of the hand. It is a normal reflex in infants up to about 5 months of age but is a pathological reflex in adults.

Gross motor functions   Those motor abilities that are performed mainly by using the proximal muscles and which allow for sitting, standing, walking, and movements of the head.

Gustatory   Relating to the sense of taste.

Gyrus   The convolutions making up the surface of the brain.

H

Hallucination   A perception that occurs without an associated stimulus to cause it.

Handedness   The preferential use of one hand to perform unimanual tasks for which either hand would do.

Headache   Pain in the head of numerous varieties. Common in cerebrovascular disease occurring not only with hemorrhage, but also with thrombosis, arterial dissections, and embolism.

Hemangioblastoma   A benign, slowly growing tumor composed of abnormal blood vessels usually occurring in the cerebellum or spinal cord of adults.

Hematomyelia   Hemorrhage into the spinal cord especially involving the gray matter.

Hematuria   A condition in which the urine contains blood or red blood cells.

Hemianopsia (Hemianopia)   Loss of vision in one-half the visual field of each eye.

Hemiballismus (Hemiballism)   Sudden, violent, flinging involuntary movements of an arm or leg on one side due to a lesion of the subthalamic nucleus.

Hemiparesis   Weakness (slight paralysis) of one side of the body.

Hemiplegia   Paralysis (severe weakness) of one side of the body.

Hemiplegic gait   The leg is held stiffly and does not flex at the hip, knee, or ankle. The leg rotates outward to describe a semicircle, first away from and then toward the trunk (circumduction). The foot scrapes the floor. The arm is carried in a flexed position.

Hemisensory syndrome   Numbness occurring unilaterally in the face, arm, and leg without other complaints. Often caused by a lacune in the internal capsule.

Hemispatial neglect   A condition in which objects or events on one side (usually the left), including that half of the patient herself, are ignored to a variable degree. Usually results from a lesion involving the right parietal lobe.

Hemisphere   One-half of the cerebrum.

Hemorrhage   The escape of blood through a ruptured vessel wall.

Hemorrhagic infarction   An infarction in which red blood cells are present in the infarcted tissue.

Heparin   A chemical that acts as an anticoagulant.

Hepatic   Relating to the liver.

Hereditary   Transmitted from parent to offspring.

Herniation   Abnormal protrusion of a part of the brain outside its normal boundaries.

High Density Lipoprotein (HDL)   A compound consisting of lipid and protein that transports cholesterol from body tissues to the liver. High levels of HDLs are considered *good* because the transported cholesterol is destined for degradation by the liver.

Hippocampus   A submerged gyrus making up the medial wall of the temporal lobe. It functions in memory.

Hoffman reflex   Reflex flexion of the fingers and thumb in response to stretch of the flexor digitorum profundus muscle.

Homonymous   The same on the two sides of the body.

Homunculus   A caricature of the body overlying the primary motor and sensory cortices of a hemisphere that shows the area of cortex containing the representation of each body part.

Horizontal gaze palsy   Inability to turn the eyes conjugately to one side caused by a lesion to the pons on the same side or to the frontal lobe on the opposite side.

Horner Syndrome   Meiosis, ptosis, and decreased sweating due to a lesion at any point in the sympathetic pathway.

Hydrocephalus   A condition characterized by the excessive accumulation of cerebrospinal fluid in the ventricles of the brain with a resultant thinning of brain tissues.

Hyperesthesia Increased sensitivity to touch, pain, or other sensory stimuli often with an added unpleasant quality.

Hypermetria An excessive range of movement of a limb such that the limb over-shoots its intended target. A sign of a cerebellar lesion.

Hypersomnia Excessive sleep.

Hypertension High blood pressure.

Hypertonia Increased resistance of a muscle to passive stretching as occurs in spasticity and rigidity.

Hypoglossal nerve The XIIth cranial nerve supplying the tongue muscles.

Hypotonia Decreased resistance of a muscle to passive stretching.

Hypoxia Abnormally low levels of oxygen in inspired air, arterial blood, or a tissue.

I

Iatrogenic A condition caused by a medical or surgical treatment.

Ictal A sudden neurological event such as a seizure or stroke.

Idiopathic A disease arising spontaneously with no known cause.

Illusion A distortion of on-going perception caused by an immediate environmental stimulus.

Implicit memory See **nondeclarative memory**.

Inattention Lack of attention to a sensory stimulus.

Incontinence The inadvertent or uncontrolled discharge of urine or feces or both.

Incoordination See **ataxia**.

Infarct An area of tissue necrosis due to insufficient blood supply.

Inhibit To restrain.

Insomnia The subjective feeling of a decrease in the quantity or quality of sleep.

Intelligence The capacity for knowledge and understanding, especially as applied to adjusting one's behavior to successfully handle novel situations.

Intention tremor An involuntary oscillation of a limb that worsens as it approaches a desired object.

Interictal The interval between seizures.

Internuclear ophthalmoplegia When the patient attempts to look laterally out of the corner of one eye, the other eye will not cross the midline toward the nose (will not adduct), while the eye that does move laterally (abducts) will show rhythmic jerking movements called nystagmus.

Interoception Denoting information originating from sensory receptors located within the walls of visceral organs such as the respiratory or gastrointestinal tracts.

Interstitial As applied to the brain, the fluid and neuroglial cells occupying the space between nerve cells.

Interstitial brain edema An increase in the amount of water in the extracellular space adjacent to the ventricles as a result of increased intracranial pressure.

Intracerebral hemorrhage (Intraparenchymal hemorrhage) Bleeding into the substance of the brain.

Intracranial arteries   Arteries within the skull.

Intracranial pressure   The pressure inside the skull.

Intramedullary   Situated within the spinal cord or brain stem.

Intraventricular hemorrhage   Bleeding into the ventricles of the brain.

Involuntary movements   Abnormal, spontaneous movements that are not under voluntary control.

Ischemia   Local anemia due to mechanical obstruction of the arterial supply.

Ischemic infarction   Necrosis of brain tissue due to ischemia.

Ischemic penumbra   The zone surrounding an infarct in which the cells are inactive but still viable. When perfusion is restored, the cells will become functional once again. The zone surrounding an infarct where the damage is reversible.

J

Jamais vu   Feeling of strangeness or unfamiliarity.

Jaw jerk reflex   A downward tap on the examiner's finger which is placed on the patient's chin elicits contraction of the masseter and temporalis (jaw closing) muscles.

Joint position sense (Conscious proprioception)   The capacity to determine the position of a body part without the use of vision.

K

Kinesthesis   The capacity to discriminate the movement of a body part and its direction without the use of vision.

Knee jerk (Patellar reflex, Quadriceps reflex, Tendon jerk reflex)   Contraction of the quadriceps muscle and extension of the knee when the patellar tendon is tapped with a reflex hammer.

Korsakoff Syndrome (Korsakoff psychosis)   A mental disorder in which the inability to record new information (loss of anterograde, or recent, memory) is impaired out of proportion to other cognitive capacities in an otherwise alert, responsive patient. Confabulation may be present but is an inconsistent symptom. Due to lesions in the medial temporal lobes or dorsomedial thalamus.

L

Labyrinth   The inner ear consisting of the cochlea (for hearing), and the vestibule and semicircular canals (for balance, equilibrium).

Lacunar state   The presence of multiple small infarcts in the white matter, which, when the necrotic tissue has been removed, leave behind small cavities called lacunes. The lacunar state may result in a pure motor hemiplegia or a pure hemisensory syndrome.

Lacune   A small cavity in the white matter of the brain, brain stem, or cerebellum resulting from occlusion of deep penetrating arterioles.

Lancinating pain   A sharp cutting or tearing pain resembling that of a stab with a needle or scalpel.

Language disorder   Disturbances in reading, writing, spelling, verbal learning and memory, and aphasia.

Latency   The length of time intervening between a stimulus or exposure to an event and the occurrence of a response.

Latent   Concealed, not yet manifest, but potentially observable.

Lateral inferior pontine syndrome   Deafness, facial palsy, facial numbness, and cerebellar ataxia due to a small pontine vascular lesion.

Lateral medullary syndrome (Wallenberg Syndrome, syndrome of the posterior inferior cerebellar artery)   Dysarthria, dysphagia, hoarseness, vertigo, oscillopsia, ataxia, Horner Syndrome, and loss of pain and temperature on the ipsilateral side of the face and contralateral side of the body (alternating thermoanalgesia) due to occlusion of the vertebral artery or its branch, the posterior inferior cerebellar artery.

Lateralization   Localization of a cerebral function to one or the other of the cerebral hemispheres.

Leptomeninges   The pia mater and arachnoid, which together enclose CSF.

Lethargy   An imprecise term sometimes applied to a state of impaired consciousness from which the patient can be aroused.

Light reflex   Reflex constriction of both pupils when light is shown in one eye. The term *direct* is applied to the reflex elicited in the stimulated eye, and *consensual* to the reflex elicited in the nonstimulated eye.

Limbic system   The structures considered as parts of the limbic system vary, depending on who lists them. The functions of the system are not completely understood, but include smell, emotion, and memory.

Lipohyalinosis   The pathological change in intracerebral arteries of patients with hypertensive vascular disease.

Lobar hemorrhage   Bleeding into the cerebrum outside the basal ganglia.

Localization   The idea that specific functions are located in different parts of the brain. A cortical function in which the site of a stimulus is referred to a specific site on the body.

Locked-in syndrome   A state in which an aware patient is unable to respond adequately due to a near total motor paralysis. The patient is mute and akinetic, but can respond by moving his eyes or eyelids. A major lesion of the pons with basilar artery occlusion produces the syndrome.

Low Density Lipoprotein (LDL)   A compound consisting of lipid and protein that transports cholesterol to the peripheral tissues making it available for membrane or hormone synthesis and for storage for later use. High LDL levels are considered *bad* because excessive LDL levels result in cholesterol deposits in the cells of artery walls.

Lower motor neuron   Neurons whose cell bodies are located within the central nervous system and whose axons innervate striated (voluntary) muscle.

Lumbar puncture   An invasive procedure in which a needle is inserted between the 4th and 5th lumbar vertebrae into the subarachnoid space for the purpose of obtaining a sample of cerebrospinal fluid.

M

Macular sparing   The condition in a patient with homonymous hemianopsia wherein the macular representation in the cortex is spared leaving an island of central vision in a sea of blindness.

Magnetic resonance imaging (MRI)   A technique that provides slice images of the brain in any plane. MRI measures the activity of the nuclei of hydrogen atoms in the brain by placing the body in a strong magnetic field and then exciting the nuclei with bursts of radiofrequency energy.

Malingering   The conscious, motivated feigning of illness or disability.

Mass lesions   Pathological accumulations of foreign material inside the cranium that act to dramatically increase intracranial pressure.

Mass reflex   Flexor muscle spasms and autonomic discharge after the period of spinal shock in patients suffering from complete or near-complete damage to the spinal cord.

Mathew scale   A scoring system used for the evaluation of stroke patients.

Medial lemniscus   The fiber tract (bundle of axons) that carries discriminative sensory information through the brain stem into the thalamus.

Medial medullary syndrome   A brain stem syndrome resulting from occlusion of the paramedian branches of the vertebral artery. The syndrome consists of ipsilateral paralysis and atrophy of the tongue, contralateral paralysis of the arm and leg, and contralateral loss of position and vibration sense.

Medulla oblongata (medulla)   The part of the brain stem between the pons and spinal cord.

Medullary   Relating to the medulla or marrow.

Medullary pyramid   The fiber tract (bundle of axons) in the medulla that carries information from the cerebral cortex that is used to control voluntary movement.

Medullary respiratory centers   Groups of nerve cells in the medulla that function as a pattern generator for respiration.

Memory   The capacity to retain and recall that which was once learned or experienced.

Meninges   The membranous coverings of the central nervous system consisting of the dura mater, arachnoid, and pia mater.

Meningitis   Inflammation of the meninges of the brain or spinal cord by bacterial, viral, or fungal infectious agents, or as a result of toxic agents or tumors.

Mesencephalon   See **midbrain**.

Meyers loop   A component of the visual radiation from the thalamus to the occipital lobe that is present in the anterior temporal lobe. It contains fibers from the inferior nasal quadrants of the retina, which when damaged produce a "pie in the sky" visual deficit in each eye.

Micturition   Urination.

Midbrain   The **mesencephalon**. That portion of the brain stem between the pons and thalamus.

Migraine stroke   Migrainous symptoms (scintillating scotomas, blurred vision, blindness, numbness, paresthesia, aphasia, dysarthria, motor weakness) that are not fully reversible within seven days associated with neuroimaging confirmation of ischemic infarction.

Miosis   Constriction of the pupil.

Modality   A type of sensation such as pain, temperature, touch, pressure, vibration, position, or movement or one of the special senses.

Monocular   Relating to one eye.

Monoplegia   Paralysis of a single limb.

Morbid   Diseased or pathologic.

Motility   The power of spontaneous movement.

Motor aphasia   See **Broca's aphasia**.

Motor cortex   Those areas of the cerebral cortex devoted to the control of movement.

Motor disorders   Impairments of motor function including paralysis, involuntary movements, and apraxias.

MRI   See **magnetic resonance imaging**.

Multifocal   As applied to disorders of the nervous system, a pathological process occurring in numerous, separate sites of the nervous system with signs and symptoms referable to those sites.

Multi-infarct dementia   Deterioration of mental functions and behavior resulting from many usually relatively small infarcts of the brain.

Muscle atrophy   Reduction in the number or size of muscle cells due to disease or disuse.

Muscle fatigue   The inability to maintain force.

Muscle power   The ability to generate force.

Muscle sense   An old term for *position sense* (proprioception) and the *sense of movement* (kinesthesia).

Muscle stretch reflex   Reflex contraction of a muscle in response to its sudden lengthening.

Muscle tone   The resistance of muscle to passive lengthening.

Mutism   Absence of the faculty of speech.

Mydriasis   Dilation of the pupils due to paresis or paralysis of smooth muscles of the iris.

Myelin   The fatty material forming an insulating sheath around the axons of some nerve cells and increasing the speed of conduction of the action potential along the axon.

Myelination   The process of formation of the myelin sheath investing axons.

Myelitis   Inflammation of the substance of the spinal cord.

Myocardial infarction   Infarction of an area of heart muscle usually as a result of occlusion of a coronary artery.

Myoclonus   Sudden, involuntary contractions of a muscle or muscle groups due to hyperexcitability of the nervous system.

Myopathy   A disease affecting the structure and function of muscle.

Myopia   Nearsightedness; shortsightedness.

Myotasis   Stretching of a muscle.

Myotatic   Relating to myotasis.

Myotatic reflexes   Muscle stretch reflexes.

N

Narcolepsy   A disorder of sudden uncontrollable episodes of sleep occurring at irregular intervals in the absence of predisposing causes.

Near point   The closest point in front of the eyes at which an object is still in focus.

Neck rigidity   Increased stiffness of the neck muscles to flexion of the neck due to irritation of the meninges from any cause.

Necrosis   Irreversible destruction of the cells of a tissue.

Negative symptoms   Functional deficits caused by the loss of capacities controlled by the damaged structure.

Neglect   A condition in which sensory events in the contralateral (usually left) half of extrapersonal space have little or no impact upon awareness.

Neocerebellum   That portion of the cerebellum controlling voluntary movement consisting of most of the cerebellar hemispheres.

Neocortex   By far the largest part of the human cerebral cortex consisting of cells arranged in six layers.

Neologism   A newly created word without conventional meaning.

Neonatal   Relating to the period from immediately after birth through the first 28 days of life.

Neoplasm   A tumor consisting of an abnormal proliferation of brain cells, which may be benign or malignant (cancer).

Nerve   A bundle of axons and its supporting connective tissue present in the peripheral nervous system and by which stimuli are conducted from the central nervous system to a body part or the reverse.

Neural   Relating to any structure composed of nerve cells or their processes.

Neuralgia   Pain, usually severe, in the territory supplied by a nerve.

Neuritic plaques   Discrete spherical lesions averaging about 30 micrometers in diameter occurring profusely in the brains of patients with Alzheimer's disease but also present in smaller numbers in the elderly. They consist of a central core of beta-amyloid surrounded by degenerating neurites with an outer margin of reactive glial cells.

Neuritis   Inflammation of peripheral nerves from any cause.

Neurofibrillary tangles Bundles of abnormal fibrous proteins that fill the cell bodies of neurons in the brains of patients with Alzheimer's disease. Because of their arrangement, the abnormal bundles are termed *paired helical filaments.*

Neurogenic Originating in, starting from, or caused by the nervous system.

Neuroglia The cells of the nervous system that support, both structurally and metabolically, the nerve cells. Neuroglia consist of astrocytes, oligodendrocytes, microglia, and ependymal cells.

Neurologist A physician trained to diagnose and manage patients with diseases of the nervous system.

Neurology The branch of medical science concerned with the study of the nervous system and its disorders.

Neuroma A general term for a tumor (neoplasm) derived from cells of the nervous system.

Neuron A nerve cell and its processes.

Neuropathy A disease involving the cranial or spinal nerves.

Neuropil The complex, feltlike net of the processes of neurons and glial cells within which are embedded the cell bodies of neurons.

Neurotomy The surgical cutting of a nerve.

Neurotransmitter A chemical synthesized and stored in a nerve cell, which when released onto another cell causes the receiving cell to respond.

Neurovascular syndromes The clinical picture that results from occlusion of a given cerebral artery.

NMR Acronym for *nuclear magnetic resonance* but now referred to as ***magnetic resonance imaging***.

Nociceptive Capable of receiving or transmitting pain.

Nociceptive reflex The family of reflexes elicited by painful stimuli.

Nociceptor A receptor in body periphery that responds to tissue injury.

Noncommunicating hydrocephalus A poor term designating a form of hydrocephalus in which cerebrospinal fluid does not drain from the ventricles into the subarachnoid space. Also termed *obstructive* or *internal hydrocephalus.*

Nondeclarative memory The capacity to learn a complex skill (performance) without being aware of the specific events that allow the person to learn the rules and procedures that make up the skill. An example is learning how to draw by looking at your hand in a mirror.

Nonfluency Effortful speech that exhibits dysprosodia.

Nonfluent aphasia See **Broca's aphasia**.

Nuchal rigidity Stiffness of the neck that may be a sign of intracerebral hemorrhage.

Numbness The absence of the perception of touch, temperature, or pain.

Nucleus ambiguus The group of cell bodies in the brain stem that regulate the contractions of the muscles of the pharynx and larynx and thus participate in such functions as swallowing and making voiced speech sounds.

Nystagmus   Rhythmical, conjugate deviations of the eyes consisting of slow and fast phases.

O

Obtundation   A reduced level of consciousness from which the patient can be roused with verbal or painful stimuli during the period of stimulation.

Occipital lobes   The paired posterior lobes of the brain concerned with visual functions.

Occlusion   The act of a hollow structure, such as an artery, closing or the state of being closed.

Occult   Hidden, concealed, not manifest.

Ocular bobbing   A spontaneous fast jerk of both eyes in a downward direction, followed by a slow drift to the midposition most often associated with a large lesion to the pons, sometimes with a lesion to the cerebellum.

Oculomotor nerve   The third cranial nerve supplying somatic motor fibers to all the extraocular muscles except the lateral rectus and superior oblique and parasympathetic motor fibers controlling pupillary constriction.

Oligodendroglia   Supporting cells of the brain and spinal cord whose processes form the myelin sheaths investing axons of the central nervous system.

One-and-a-half syndrome   A disorder of eye movement characterized by the patient's inability to move either eye toward the side of the lesion (the "one") in lateral gaze, or to move the eye on the side of the lesion in gaze toward the opposite side (the "half").

Ophthalmoplegia   Paralysis of one or more of the extraocular eye muscles resulting in abnormal eye movements.

Ophthalmoscope   An instrument for examining the interior of the eye through the pupil.

Opisthotonos   Strong extensor muscle contractions resulting, when the patient is lying supine, in the body resting on the back of the head and heels due to a severe midbrain lesion.

Optic ataxia   A failure to touch or grasp an object when the movement is guided by vision due to bilateral occipital lobe lesions. A component of the Balint Syndrome.

Optic neuritis   Inflammation of the optic nerve due to various causes.

Orgogozo scale   A simple method of estimating the deficits suffered by patients with stroke.

Orthostatic hypotension   A reduction in arterial blood pressure on assuming an erect posture.

Oscillopsia   The illusion of the rhythmic oscillation of objects in the environment.

P

Pain   The unpleasant sensation associated with actual or potential tissue damage.

Pale infarction   Infarcts that have no blood and therefore are pale.

Paleocerebellum   The anterior lobe of the cerebellum.

Palsy   Lack of power, paralysis, or paresis.

Papilledema   Swelling of the optic nerve head as a result of increased intracranial pressure.

Paralysis   Loss of the power of voluntary movement.

Paramagnetic agents   Chemical substances, which when injected into a patient increase the quality of the images produced by magnetic resonance imaging. See **gadolinium.**

Paraparesis   Weakness of the legs.

Paraphasia   A process of substitution in which one sound (phoneme) or syllable in a word is substituted for the correct one (*literal paraphasia*), in which an incorrect word is substituted for the correct word (*verbal paraphasia*), or in which a meaningless set of sounds is substituted for the correct word (*neologism*). A manifestation of Wernicke's aphasia.

Paraplegia   Paralysis of the legs.

Parasympathetic nervous system   The division of the autonomic nervous system responsible for activities that lower the metabolic rate and restore and conserve energy.

Parenchyma   The cells that actually make up an organ, such as the brain, as distinguished from the cells that structurally support the organ (the stroma).

Paresis   A weakness in the power of voluntary movement.

Paretic   Of or relating to a paresis.

Paresthesias   Abnormal sensations such as tingling, burning, or pricking.

Parietal lobe   The lobe of the cerebral hemisphere posterior to the frontal lobe, anterior to the occipital lobe, and superior to the temporal lobe.

Parkinsonism   A brain disorder characterized by a classic triad of neurological signs including resting tremor, akinesia (bradykinesia) and muscular rigidity. Due to interference with dopamine-mediated neurotransmission in the basal ganglia caused by degeneration of neurons in the substantia nigra or antipsychotic medication.

Parkinsonism-plus   A group of disorders in which parkinsonism is accompanied by signs of other disorders, for example, pyramidal signs or cerebellar signs.

Paroxysm   The sudden onset of a symptom such as a sharp spasm or convulsion.

Paroxysmal   Occurring in paroxysms.

Past pointing   The condition in which a patient, in attempting to touch a target with his finger, fails to come to a stop when the target is reached. A sign of cerebellar disease.

Patellar reflex   See **knee jerk**.

Pathological crying   Involuntary crying in response to an inappropriate stimulus, a result of bilateral lesions to the internal capsule.

Pathological laughter   Involuntary laugher in response to an inappropriate stimulus, a result of bilateral lesions of the internal capsule.

Pedal   Relating to the foot.

Peduncle   A neuroanatomical term applied to stalk-like structures that connect two parts of the brain, such as the *cerebral peduncles* of the midbrain or the *cerebellar peduncles* that connect the cerebellum to different parts of the brain stem.

Pendular knee jerk   A knee jerk reflex in which the leg swings back and forth a greater number of times than normal, due to hypotonia caused by cerebellar lesions.

Perception   The process of becoming aware of or recognizing an object including its significance and emotional meaning.

Perfusion pressure   The difference between the mean arterial pressure and intracranial pressure (cerebral venous pressure).

Perimetry   The mapping of visual fields.

Periventricular   Neural tissue surrounding the ventricles of the brain.

Perseveration   The repetition of an activity without an appropriate stimulus.

Persistent vegetative state   A condition that follows a deep coma in which the patient's eyes are open but he is unconscious, unaware of himself or his environment. Brain stem functions such as breathing, swallowing, chewing, and cranial nerve reflexes are preserved.

PET scan   A technique for showing the regional metabolism of nerve cells in the brain. See **positron emission tomography**.

Phantom limb   The subjective perception (often painful) of the presence of a limb when it is absent either congenitally or due to amputation.

Phonation   The generation of sounds by the larynx.

Physical therapy   The treatment of neurologic deficits, pain, and injury by physical means.

Pia mater   The innermost of the three meninges, firmly adherent to the surface of the brain and spinal cord.

Pill-rolling tremor   See **resting tremor**.

Plantar reflex   Normal flexion of the toes resulting from stimulation of the sole of the foot.

Pleocytosis   Presence of more cells than normal.

Polycythemia vera   An increase above normal in the number of red cells in the blood. The resultant high blood viscosity, engorgement of vessels, and reduced rate of blood flow cause a high incidence of thrombosis.

Pons   The portion of the brain stem between the medulla and the midbrain.

Pontine hemorrhage   Primary intracerebral hemorrhage into the pons usually producing deep coma in a few minutes and characterized clinically by total paralysis and small pupils that react to light.

Positive symptoms   Positive symptoms involve an excess of neural activity and the expenditure of energy. They are due to overactivity of undamaged parts of the nervous system.

Positron emission tomography (PET)   A technique for imaging the brain that measures the cerebral concentration in different brain areas of systemically administered radioactive tracers.

Posterior cerebral artery syndromes   Syndromes resulting from the occlusion of the posterior cerebral artery by a thrombus or embolism.

Posterior thalamic syndrome   See **thalamic syndrome**.

Postictal state   The period of depressed neurological function lasting minutes or hours that follows the occurrence of a seizure.

Postural reflexes   Patterns of involuntary muscle contractions designed to compensate for shifts in the position of the body in relation to the line of gravity.

Praxis   The performance of an action, as of a manual task.

Prefrontal cortex   The parts of the frontal lobe rostral to the primary motor and premotor cortices whose destruction leads to disorders such as loss of recent memory, insight and foresight, and to indifference and euphoria.

Primary (hypertensive) intracerebral hemorrhage   Bleeding within brain tissue as a result of the rupture of an artery due to hypertension.

Primary motor area   The area of the cerebral cortex, comprising the precentral gyrus, or Brodmann's area 4, that controls voluntary movements of the opposite half of the body.

Primary sensory area   The area of the cerebral cortex, comprising the postcentral gyrus, or Brodmann's areas 3, 1, and 2, that first receives sensation from the body **(somatic sensation)**.

Priapism   Prolonged, painful erection sometimes resulting from antipsychotic or antidepressant medication, or from spinal cord lesions.

Procedural memory   See **nondeclarative memory**.

Prodrome   A symptom providing early warning of a disease.

Progressive   Denoting the worsening course of a disease.

Pronation-supination test   The patient is required to perform rapid alternating rotatory movements of the forearm, first pronating then supinating the forearm on the knee. Patients with damage to the cerebellum have difficulty performing this test. See **adiadochokinesis**.

Propositional language   Learned, symbolic language used to communicate ideas from one person to another, as distinguished from emotional language.

Proprioception   Denoting information originating from sensory receptors in muscles, tendons, joints, and other deep tissues of the body. Also, the capacity to locate the position of the limbs in space.

Prosody   The melodious aspect of speech with an emphasis on stress, rhythm, and intonation by which both linguistic and affective information is conveyed. Broca's aphasics suffer from *dysprosody,* an impairment in prosody.

Prosopagnosia   A failure to recognize familiar faces caused by bilateral lesions in the inferior occipitotemporal lobes.

Pseudo   False.

Pseudobulbar palsy   Spastic weakness or paralysis of voluntary movements of the jaw, face, tongue, larynx, and pharynx often occurring with pathologic laughing and crying as a result of bilateral lesions of the internal capsule. The signs and symptoms resemble those occurring in (true) bulbar palsy.

Psychogenic Originating in or caused by the mind.

Psychosis A category of mental illness defined by a gross distortion of reality and loss of reality testing. Characterized by such features.

Ptosis Drooping of the upper eyelid.

Pupil The aperture of the eye through which light passes, surrounded by the iris.

Pupillary light reflex Constriction of the pupils in response to light stimulation.

Pure alexia See **alexia without agraphia**.

Pure motor hemiplegia Paralysis or paresis of the face, arm, and leg on one side without sensory or other deficits. See **lacunar state**.

Pure Hemisensory Syndrome (pure sensory stroke) Numbness occurring on one side of the face, arm, and leg without other deficits. See **lacunar state**.

Pure word blindness See **alexia without agraphia**.

Pursuit movements Deviations of the eyes performed in order to maintain fixation upon a moving object.

Putamen A nucleus of the basal ganglia.

Putaminal hemorrhage Hemorrhage into the putamen and adjacent internal capsule usually as a result of hypertension.

Pyramidal tract Those axons that travel longitudinally through the pyramids of the medulla and control voluntary movements.

Q

Quadrantanopia Loss of vision in one-quarter of the visual field. *Superior quadrantanopia* results from temporal lobe lesions, while *inferior quadrantanopia* results from parietal lobe lesions.

Quadriplegia (tetraplegia) Paralysis of all four limbs.

Quality of life index Various attempts to formally assess the ability of a patient to successfully carry out the activities of daily living and to participate in pursuits that provide pleasure and fulfillment.

R

Radioactive isotopes An isotope with an unstable nuclear composition that regains stability by spontaneously emitting gamma rays. Used to visualize lesions of the brain.

Radiography Examination of a part of the body by means of x-rays impressed on photographic film.

Receptive aphasia See **Wernicke's aphasia**.

Radiosurgery Shooting multiple radiation beams at a target from many different directions.

Reflex A stereotyped involuntary contraction of muscles set into motion by a peripheral stimulus.

Reflex incontinence The passage of urine due to contraction of the bladder in response to stretching of the bladder wall when full.

Regeneration   The reconstitution (regrowth) of the part of the axon severed (disconnected) from the cell body of a nerve cell.

Rehabilitation   Restoration of the ability to function, partially or completely, following injury or disease.

Remission   A lessening in severity of the signs and symptoms of a disease. Remission may be spontaneous or occur following treatment. A frequent characteristic of multiple sclerosis.

Resting tremor   Involuntary contractions of antagonistic muscle groups in a distal body part occurring in the absence of voluntary movement, while the extremity is at rest.

Reticular activating system   That portion of the brain stem reticular formation that when active desynchronizes (activates) the entire cerebral cortex.

Reticular formation   The central core of the brain stem consisting of an interlacing net of neuronal processes and cell bodies with no readily apparent structural organization.

Retrograde amnesia   Loss of memory for remote events that occurred before the time of brain injury.

Rigidity   Increased resistance of muscle to passive stretching throughout the range of movement.

Romberg test   A supposed test of conscious proprioception wherein the patient stands with feet together, head erect, and the amount of body sway with the eyes open and closed is compared. When there is a tendency to fall with the eyes closed, the patient is said to have a *positive Romberg sign.*

S

Saccades   Rapid voluntary eye movements that change ocular fixation.

Saccular (berry) aneurysm   A circumscribed dilation of an artery, most often in relation to the circle of Willis at the base of the brain.

Scanning speech   Words are broken up into syllables so that speech sounds disjointed as when a line of poetry is scanned for meter.

Sclerosis   A localized area of hardness in the brain or spinal cord due to the hyperplasia of astrocytes and the formation of a glial "scar."

Scotoma   An isolated area within the visual field of varying size and shape in which vision is absent or diminished.

Segmental   An anatomical term referring to the spinal cord.

Seizure   The sudden onset of a combination of motor, sensory, or psychic events due to a sudden and excessive discharge of brain neurons. A symptom of abnormal function in the central nervous system rather than a disease in itself.

Seizure focus   The nerve cells in a small area of the cerebral cortex (usually) whose normal interrelationships have been disrupted so that they discharge electrical signals at an excessively high rate and in an abnormal pattern.

Semicoma   An imprecise term denoting a mild degree of coma from which the patient can be aroused.

Senile   When used alone, a vague term of little clinical value.

Senile plaques   Microscopic lesions present profusely in the brains of patients with Alzheimer's disease and occurring in two basic forms: the diffuse plaque and the neuritic plaque. Senile plaques are present in lesser numbers in the brains of the elderly.

Sensorimotor stroke   A syndrome in which hemiparesis is associated with hypoesthesia on one side of the body.

Sensory aphasia   See **Wernicke's aphasia**.

Sensory ataxia   Incoordinated, awkward voluntary movements as a result of the loss of proprioception.

Sensory end-organ   The specialization of the peripheral terminal of a sensory axon and/or its association with nonneural cells that render the axon terminal specifically sensitive to one type of stimulus energy and insensitive to others.

Sensory modalities   The different sensory perceptions such as pain, temperature, touch, pressure, vibration, position, and movement.

Sensory system   The pathways that carry information to the brain informing the organism about the status of its internal and external environments.

Sequela (pl. sequelae)   A condition resulting from a disease.

Short-term memory   The mental problems a person is currently working on.

Sign   An abnormality discoverable on examination indicative of a disease.

Sinistral   Denoting a left-handed person.

Simultagnosia   The inability to recognize more than one object in a particular sensory channel at one time.

Single-photon emission computed tomography (SPECT)   A technique of measuring neural activity by measuring regional changes in cerebral blood flow. The technique involves the intravenous injection of gamma-emitting isotopes, a ring of gamma-detectors, and computer reconstructions of brain slices showing active and inactive areas.

Slit hemorrhage   Bleeding into the brain at the junction of the white and gray matter due to hypertension.

Smooth pursuit movements   A reflex by which the eyes track a moving target in order to keep the image of the target on the fovea.

Snout reflex (sucking reflex)   Bilateral contraction of the lips elicited by sweeping the end of a tongue blade lightly over the lips.

Somatic sensation   Sensations that arise in the skin, muscles, and joints.

Somatotopic localization   The representation of given parts of the body within particular areas of the central nervous system.

Somesthesia   Conscious awareness of the body.

Sommer sector   A part of the hippocampus in which the pyramidal cells are especially sensitive to oxygen deprivation.

Spasm   Involuntary contractions of muscle.

Spasmodic crying   See **pathological crying**.

Spasmodic laughter   See **pathological laughter**.

Spastic paraplegia   Spastic paralysis of the legs.

Spasticity   A state of increased muscle tone with exaggerated stretch reflexes.

Spatial neglect   Lack of awareness of one-half of visual space, usually the left half, following lesions in the posterior parts of the right cerebral hemisphere.

Speech   The use of the voice and verbal symbols in the expression of thoughts and feelings.

Splenium   The posterior portion of the corpus callosum.

Stasis   Stagnation of the blood.

Status   A state or condition of longer than normal duration.

Stenosis   Pathologic narrowing of a blood vessel or other hollow viscus.

Stereoanesthesia   The lack of recognition of shape or form by handling.

Stereognosis   The appreciation of the form of an object by manipulation without the use of vision.

Strabismus   Crossed eyes.

Stress   Reactions of the body to mental or physical conditions that disturb the body's equilibrium (homeostasis).

Stretch reflex   The reflex contraction of a muscle in response to its sudden stretching by tapping on its tendon with a reflex hammer.

Striate cortex   The area of the cerebral cortex at the occipital pole that receives input from the retina.

Striatum   The caudate nucleus, putamen, and globus pallidus of the cerebrum.

Stroke   A generic term denoting a sudden, focal neurological deficit secondary to cerebral arterial or venous disease.

Stroke-in-evolution   The portion of a stroke during which the signs and symptoms increase in severity with time.

Stupor   A state of reduced consciousness in which the patient shows a marked reduction in his reaction to environmental stimuli but may make motor, but not verbal, responses to strong stimulation.

Subarachnoid hemorrhage   Bleeding into the subarachnoid space usually as a result of the rupture of a berry aneurysm.

Subcortical   Referring to any part of the brain located beneath the cerebral cortex.

Subcortical aphasia   Variable forms of aphasia resulting from infarctions in the neostriatum and thalamus.

Subdural hematoma   The accumulation of venous blood beneath the dura mater as a result of trauma.

Superficial reflexes   Reflex muscle contractions elicited by stimulating cutaneous receptors.

Supination   The position of the body when lying with the face and arms upward.

Sympathetic nervous system   The division of the autonomic nervous system concerned with increasing the rate of metabolism, energy expenditure, and alertness and responsible for the "fight or flight" response.

Symptom   An abnormal function or sensation experienced by the patient and indicative of disease.

Symptomatic   Indicative of a condition or disease.

Synapse   The specialized site of apposition at which one nerve cell transmits information to another nerve cell.

Syndrome   A collection of signs and symptoms characteristic of a particular disease.

Synergy   The coordinated action of two or more structures.

T

Tactile   Of or relating to the sense of touch.

Tactile agnosia   An inability to recognize an object by touch in either hand due to a lesion of the posterior parietal lobe of the dominant hemisphere.

Tactile discrimination   The ability to identify and quantitate stimuli applied to the skin without the use of vision. Tests of two-point discrimination, direction of a moving tactile stimulus, and traced figure identification are used to assess this capacity.

Telangiectasia   Congenital dilation of small blood vessels and capillaries.

Telegraphic speech   Aphasic speech in which substantive words are retained (nouns and verbs) and relational, filler words (articles, conjunctions, adverbs) are omitted.

Tetraplegia   See **quadriplegia**.

Thalamic hemorrhage   Bleeding into the thalamus due to rupture of branches of the posterior cerebral artery in hypertensive patients. Contralateral sensory loss and hemiparesis or hemiplegia are characteristic.

Thalamic syndrome   Unilateral facial pain and dysesthesia, transitory contralateral hemiparesis, and contralateral loss of both deep and superficial sensation due to occlusion of the penetrating branches of the posterior cerebral artery.

Thiamin   Thiamine. Vitamin B_1.

Thrombosis   Occlusion of a blood vessel by the formation of a blood clot.

Thrombus   A clot in the cardiovascular system formed from components of blood.

TIA   See **transient ischemic attacks**.

Tone   The resistance of muscle to passive stretch.

Tonic   A state of continuous action.

Top of the basilar syndrome   Visual, oculomotor and behavioral deficits following occlusion of branches of the posterior cerebral artery or arteries.

Torpor   A state in which the patient is unresponsive to external stimuli and is inactive.

Transcortical motor aphasia   Limited spontaneous speech, intact repetition, normal articulation, and good auditory comprehension due to a lesion in the subcortical white matter of the frontal lobe.

Transient ischemic attacks (TIAs) TIAs can reflect the involvement (almost always thrombotic) of any intracerebral artery or of the internal carotid artery and cause reversible ischemia in the area supplied by the artery. TIAs last for a few seconds up to 24 hours and are characterized by episodes of neurological dysfunction.

Transient monocular blindness See **amaurosis fugax**.

Tremor Involuntary rhythmic oscillations of a body part produced by alternating contractions of antagonistic muscles.

Trephining Surgical opening of the skull.

Two-point discrimination The ability to discriminate two points of simultaneous stimulation on the skin or mucosa.

U

Uncal herniation Downward displacement of portions of the temporal lobe (the uncus and parahippocampal gyrus) through the tentorial opening due to elevated intracranial pressure from a mass lesion.

Unconsciousness Loss of those mental activities whereby people are made aware of themselves and their environment.

Upper motor neurons Pathways that descend, either directly or indirectly, from the cerebral cortex and which control movement and posture.

V

Vascular dementia Progressive cognitive dysfunction due to thromboembolytic and other cerebrovascular diseases.

Vascular diseases Any pathological process involving blood vessels.

Vasodilator An agent that causes dilation of blood vessels.

Vasospasm Contraction of the muscular coats of an artery causing reduced blood flow through the artery.

Vasoconstriction A reduction in the diameter of arterioles due to contraction of the smooth muscles in the walls of the arterioles. Increases the resistance to blood flow through the affected vessels.

Vasodilation An increase in the diameter of arterioles due to the relaxation of smooth muscles in the wall of the arterioles. Decreases the resistance of blood flow through the affected vessels.

Vasogenic edema The most frequent type of cerebral edema caused by tumors, trauma, abscesses, and infarcts in which the blood-brain barrier breaks down resulting in excess water in the extracellular space.

Vein A blood vessel carrying blood from capillaries toward the heart.

Venous infarction Ischemic damage to a tissue resulting from impairment of its venous drainage.

Ventricles The normal cavities within the central nervous system filled with cerebrospinal fluid.

Vergence   The simultaneous turning in of both eyes to focus on a close object.

Vertebrobasilar system   One of the two major systems of arteries supplying the central nervous system. This system of arteries supplies the brain stem, the cerebellum, parts of the cerebrum, and spinal cord.

Vertigo   The sensation of rotation of the self or of the environment.

Visual agnosia   A disorder in which patients with normal visual perception fail to understand the nature or meaning of nonverbal visual stimuli that were understood previously.

Visual field   That portion of space simultaneously visible to one eye during steady fixation of the gaze.

Voluntary   Under conscious control.

W

Wada test   The intracarotid injection of amobarbital (AMYTAL) to determine the cerebral hemisphere dominant for speech. Injection on the dominant side temporarily abolishes the power of speech.

Wallenberg Syndrome   See **lateral medullary syndrome**.

Wallerian degeneration   The degeneration of that part of an axon severed from the cell body of the neuron.

Warfarin   An anticoagulant medication.

Watershed areas   The boundary zones between the territories of supply of the major cerebral arteries (anterior, middle, and posterior cerebral) at their peripheries that are most likely to suffer ischemia when cerebral perfusion diminishes.

Watershed infarcts   Infarcts that occur between the territories of supply of the major cerebral arteries.

Weber Syndrome   Unilateral third nerve palsy with contralateral hemiplegia due to a lesion in the midbrain.

Wernicke's aphasia   An aphasic disorder characterized by hyperfluency, paraphasic errors, and impaired comprehension due to a lesion of the dominant (usually left) parietotemporal lobes.

Wernicke's area   An area in the dominant hemisphere (usually left) responsible for the decoding of language.

Wernicke-Korsakoff Syndrome   A symptom complex comprising nystagmus, ophthalmoplegia, ataxia, and an inability to record new information caused by bilateral pinhead-sized hemorrhages in the mamillary bodies and in periventricular and periaqueductal gray matter as a result of thiamin deficiency in chronic alcoholics.

Word blindness   See **alexia without agraphia**.

X

Xanthochromia   A yellow discoloration of cerebrospinal fluid resulting from the breakdown of red blood cells following hemorrhage into the subarachnoid space.

INDEX